Environmental Health Criteria 196

METHANOL

First draft prepared by Dr L. Fishbein, Fairfax, Virginia, USA

Published under the joint sponsorship of the United Nations Environment Programme, the International Labour Organisation, and the World Health Organization, and produced within the framework of the Inter-Organization Programme for the Sound Management of Chemicals.

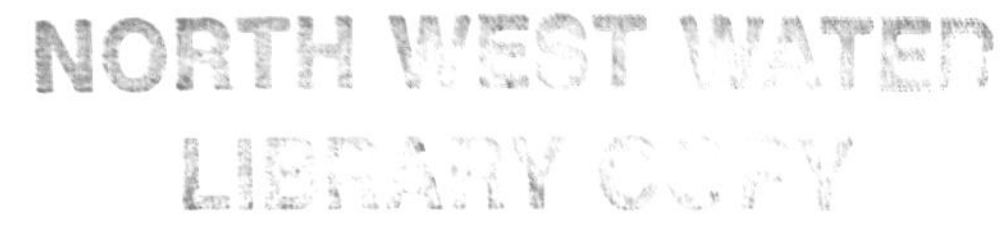

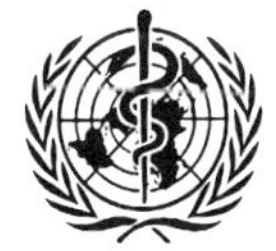

World Health Organization
Geneva, 1997

WHO Library Cataloguing in Publication Data

Methanol.

(Environmental health criteria ; 196)

1.Alcohol, Methyl - toxicity   2.Alcohol, Methyl - adverse effects
3.Environmental exposure   I.Series

ISBN 92 4 157196 9   (NLM Classification: QV 83)
ISSN 0250-863X

PRINTED IN FINLAND
97/11562 – VAMMALA – 5000

CONTENTS

ENVIRONMENTAL HEALTH CRITERIA FOR METHANOL

P R E A M B L E

Objectives

In 1973 the WHO Environmental Health Criteria Programme was initiated with the following objectives:

(i)   to assess information on the relationship between exposure to environmental pollutants and human health, and to provide guidelines for setting exposure limits;

(ii) to identify new or potential pollutants;

(iii) to identify gaps in knowledge concerning the health effects of pollutants;

(iv) to promote the harmonization of toxicological and epidemiological methods in order to have internationally comparable results.

The first Environmental Health Criteria (EHC) monograph, on mercury, was published in 1976 and since that time an ever-increasing number of assessments of chemicals and of physical effects have been produced. In addition, many EHC monographs have been devoted to evaluating toxicological methodology, e.g., for genetic, neurotoxic, teratogenic and nephrotoxic effects. Other publications have been concerned with epidemiological guidelines, evaluation of short-term tests for carcinogens, biomarkers, effects on the elderly and so forth.

Since its inauguration the EHC Programme has widened its scope, and the importance of environmental effects, in addition to health effects, has been increasingly emphasized in the total evaluation of chemicals.

The original impetus for the Programme came from World Health Assembly resolutions and the recommendations of the 1972 UN Conference on the Human Environment. Subsequently the work became an integral part of the International Programme on Chemical Safety (IPCS), a cooperative programme of UNEP, ILO and WHO. In this manner, with the strong support of the new partners, the importance of occupational health and environmental effects was fully recognized. The EHC monographs have become widely established, used and recognized throughout the world.

The recommendations of the 1992 UN Conference on Environment and Development and the subsequent establishment of the Intergovernmental Forum on Chemical Safety with the priorities for action in the six programme areas of Chapter 19, Agenda 21, all lend further weight to the need for EHC assessments of the risks of chemicals.

Scope

The criteria monographs are intended to provide critical reviews on the effect on human health and the environment of chemicals and of combinations of chemicals and physical and biological agents. As such, they include and review studies that are of direct relevance for the evaluation. However, they do not describe *every* study carried out. Worldwide data are used and are quoted from original studies, not from abstracts or reviews. Both published and unpublished reports are considered and it is incumbent on the authors to assess all the articles cited in the references. Preference is always given to published data. Unpublished data are only used when relevant published data are absent or when they are pivotal to the risk assessment. A detailed policy statement is available that describes the procedures used for unpublished proprietary data so that this information can be used in the evaluation without compromising its confidential nature (WHO (1990) Revised Guidelines for the Preparation of Environmental Health Criteria Monographs. PCS/90.69, Geneva, World Health Organization).

In the evaluation of human health risks, sound human data, whenever available, are preferred to animal data. Animal and *in vitro* studies provide support and are used mainly to supply evidence missing from human studies. It is mandatory that research on human subjects is conducted in full accord with ethical principles, including the provisions of the Helsinki Declaration.

The EHC monographs are intended to assist national and international authorities in making risk assessments and subsequent risk management decisions. They represent a thorough evaluation of risks and are not, in any sense, recommendations for regulation or standard setting. These latter are the exclusive purview of national and regional governments.

Content

The layout of EHC monographs for chemicals is outlined below.

- Summary - a review of the salient facts and the risk evaluation of the chemical
- Identity - physical and chemical properties, analytical methods
- Sources of exposure
- Environmental transport, distribution and transformation
- Environmental levels and human exposure
- Kinetics and metabolism in laboratory animals and humans
- Effects on laboratory mammals and *in vitro* test systems
- Effects on humans
- Effects on other organisms in the laboratory and field
- Evaluation of human health risks and effects on the environment
- Conclusions and recommendations for protection of human health and the environment
- Further research
- Previous evaluations by international bodies, e.g., IARC, JECFA, JMPR

Selection of chemicals

Since the inception of the EHC Programme, the IPCS has organized meetings of scientists to establish lists of priority chemicals for subsequent evaluation. Such meetings have been held in: Ispra, Italy, 1980; Oxford, United Kingdom, 1984; Berlin, Germany, 1987; and North Carolina, USA, 1995. The selection of chemicals has been based on the following criteria: the existence of scientific evidence that the substance presents a hazard to human health and/or the environment; the possible use, persistence, accumulation or degradation of the substance shows that there may be significant human or environmental exposure; the size and nature of populations at risk (both human and other species) and risks for environment;

international concern, i.e. the substance is of major interest to several countries; adequate data on the hazards are available.

If an EHC monograph is proposed for a chemical not on the priority list, the IPCS Secretariat consults with the Cooperating Organizations and all the Participating Institutions before embarking on the preparation of the monograph.

Procedures

The order of procedures that result in the publication of an EHC monograph is shown in the flow chart. A designated staff member of IPCS, responsible for the scientific quality of the document, serves as Responsible Officer (RO). The IPCS Editor is responsible for layout and language. The first draft, prepared by consultants or, more usually, staff from an IPCS Participating Institution, is based initially on data provided from the International Register of Potentially Toxic Chemicals, and reference data bases such as Medline and Toxline.

The draft document, when received by the RO, may require an initial review by a small panel of experts to determine its scientific quality and objectivity. Once the RO finds the document acceptable as a first draft, it is distributed, in its unedited form, to well over 150 EHC contact points throughout the world who are asked to comment on its completeness and accuracy and, where necessary, provide additional material. The contact points, usually designated by governments, may be Participating Institutions, IPCS Focal Points, or individual scientists known for their particular expertise. Generally some four months are allowed before the comments are considered by the RO and author(s). A second draft incorporating comments received and approved by the Director, IPCS, is then distributed to Task Group members, who carry out the peer review, at least six weeks before their meeting.

The Task Group members serve as individual scientists, not as representatives of any organization, government or industry. Their function is to evaluate the accuracy, significance and relevance of the information in the document and to assess the health and environmental risks from exposure to the chemical. A summary and

EHC PREPARATION FLOW CHART

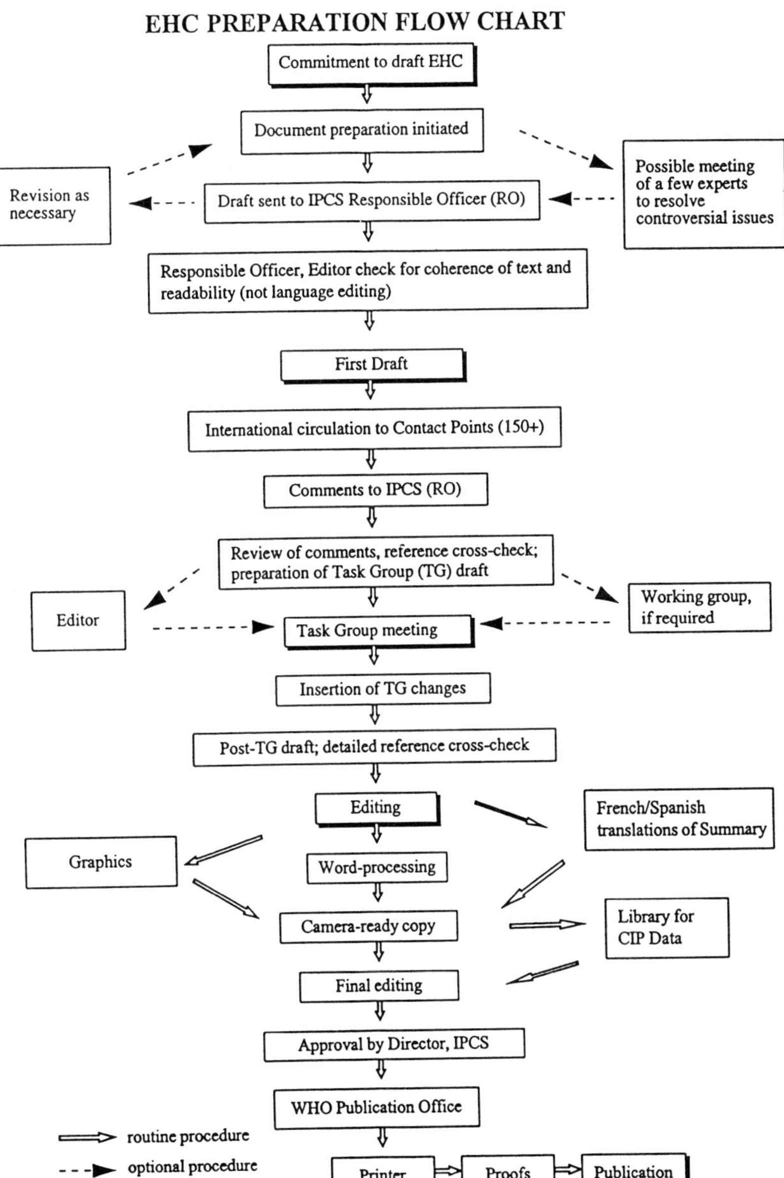

recommendations for further research and improved safety aspects are also required. The composition of the Task Group is dictated by the range of expertise required for the subject of the meeting and by the need for a balanced geographical distribution.

The three cooperating organizations of the IPCS recognize the important role played by nongovernmental organizations. Representatives from relevant national and international associations may be invited to join the Task Group as observers. While observers may provide a valuable contribution to the process, they can only speak at the invitation of the Chairperson. Observers do not participate in the final evaluation of the chemical; this is the sole responsibility of the Task Group members. When the Task Group considers it to be appropriate, it may meet *in camera*.

All individuals who as authors, consultants or advisers participate in the preparation of the EHC monograph must, in addition to serving in their personal capacity as scientists, inform the RO if at any time a conflict of interest, whether actual or potential, could be perceived in their work. They are required to sign a conflict of interest statement. Such a procedure ensures the transparency and probity of the process.

When the Task Group has completed its review and the RO is satisfied as to the scientific correctness and completeness of the document, it then goes for language editing, reference checking, and preparation of camera-ready copy. After approval by the Director, IPCS, the monograph is submitted to the WHO Office of Publications for printing. At this time a copy of the final draft is sent to the Chairperson and Rapporteur of the Task Group to check for any errors.

It is accepted that the following criteria should initiate the updating of an EHC monograph: new data are available that would substantially change the evaluation; there is public concern for health or environmental effects of the agent because of greater exposure; an appreciable time period has elapsed since the last evaluation.

All Participating Institutions are informed, through the EHC progress report, of the authors and institutions proposed for the drafting of the documents. A comprehensive file of all comments received on drafts of each EHC monograph is maintained and is available on request. The Chairpersons of Task Groups are briefed before each meeting on their role and responsibility in ensuring that these rules are followed.

WHO TASK GROUP ON ENVIRONMENTAL HEALTH CRITERIA FOR METHANOL

Members

Dr D. Anderson, British Industry Biological Research Association (BIBRA) Toxicology International, Carshalton, Surrey, United Kingdom

Dr S.A. Assimon, Contaminants Standards Monitoring and Projects Branch, US Food and Drug Administration, Washington DC, USA

Dr H.B.S. Conacher, Bureau of Chemical Safety, Ottawa, Ontario, Canada

Professor J. Eells, Department of Pharmacology and Toxicology, Medical College of Wisconsin Milwaukee, USA (*Chairman*)

Mr J. Fawell, National Centre for Environmental Toxicology, Marlow, Essex, United Kingdom

Dr L. Fishbein, Fairfax, Virginia, USA (*Joint Rapporteur*)

Dr K. McMartin, Department of Pharmacology and Therapeutics, Louisiana State University Medical Center, Shreveport, Louisiana, USA

Mr H. Malcolm, Institute of Terrestrial Ecology, Monks Wood, Huntingdon, United Kingdom (*Joint Rapporteur*)

Dr H.B. Matthews, National Institute of Environmental Health Sciences, Research Triangle Park, North Carolina, USA

Professor M. Piscator, Karolinska Institute, Stockholm, Sweden (*Vice-Chairman*)

Dr G. Rosner, Merzhausen, Germany

Representatives of other Organizations

Professor K.R. Butterworth, BIBRA Toxicology International,
Carshalton, Surrey, United Kingdom (representing the
International Union of Toxicology)

Mr M.G. Penman, ICI Chemicals & Polymers Limited,
Middlesbrough, Cleveland, United Kingdom (representing the
European Centre for Ecotoxicology and Toxicology of
Chemicals)

Secretariat

Dr E. Smith, International Programme on Chemical Safety, World
Health Organization, Geneva, Switzerland (*Secretary*)

Mr J.D. Wilbourn, Unit of Carcinogen Identification and
Evaluation, International Agency for Research on Cancer
(IARC), Lyon, France

ENVIRONMENTAL HEALTH CRITERIA FOR METHANOL

A WHO Task Group on Environmental Health Criteria for Methanol met at the British Industrial Biological Research Association (BIBRA) Toxicology International, Carshalton, Surrey, United Kingdom from 28 to 31 October 1996. Dr D. Anderson opened the meeting and welcomed the participants on behalf of the host institute. Dr E. Smith, IPCS, welcomed the participants on behalf of the Director, IPCS, and the three IPCS cooperating organizations (UNEP/ILO/WHO). The Task Group reviewed and revised the draft criteria monograph and made an evaluation of the risks for human health and the environment from exposure to methanol.

Dr L. Fishbein, Fairfax, Virginia, USA prepared the first draft of this monograph. The second draft, incorporating comments received following the circulation of the first draft to the IPCS Contact Points for Environmental Health Criteria monographs, was also prepared by Dr Fishbein.

Dr E.M. Smith and Dr P.G. Jenkins, both of the IPCS Central Unit, were responsible for the overall scientific content and technical editing, respectively.

The efforts of all who helped in the preparation and finalization of the monograph are gratefully acknowledged.

ABBREVIATIONS

ATP	adenosine triphosphate
BCF	bioconcentration factor
BOD	biochemical oxygen demand
COD	chemical oxygen demand
CNS	central nervous system
FID	flame ionization detection
GC	gas chromatography
MLD	minimum lethal dose
MS	mass spectrometry
MTBE	methyl tertiary butyl ether
NAD	nicotinamide adenine dinucleotide
NCAM	neural cell adhesion molecule
NOAEL	no-observed-adverse-effect level
THF	tetrahydrofolate
TLV	threshold limit value

1. SUMMARY

1.1 Identity, physical and chemical properties, analytical methods

Methanol is a clear, colourless, volatile flammable liquid with a mild alcoholic odour when pure. It is miscible with water and many organic solvents and forms many binary azeotropic mixtures.

Analytical methods, principally gas chromatography (GC) with flame ionization detection (FID), are available for the determination of methanol in various environmental media (air, water, soil and sediments) and foods, as well as the determination of methanol and its principal metabolite, formate, in body fluids and tissues. In addition to GC-FID, enzymatic procedures with colorimetric end-points are utilized for the determination of formate in blood, urine and tissues.

Determination of methanol in the workplace usually involves collection and concentration on silica gel, followed by aqueous extraction and GC-FID or GC-mass spectrometry analysis of the extract.

1.2 Sources of human exposure

Methanol occurs naturally in humans, animals and plants. It is a natural constituent in blood, urine, saliva and expired air. A mean urinary methanol level of 0.73 mg/litre (range 0.3-2.61 mg/litre) in unexposed individuals and a range of 0.06 to 0.32 µg/litre in expired air have been reported.

The two most important sources of background body burdens for methanol and formate are diet and metabolic processes. Methanol is available in the diet principally from fresh fruits and vegetables, fruit juices (average 140 mg/litre, range 12 to 640 mg/litre), fermented beverages (up to 1.5 g/litre) and diet foods (principally soft drinks). The artificial sweetener aspartame is widely used and, on hydrolysis, 10% (by weight) of the molecule is converted to free methanol, which is available for absorption.

About 20 million tonnes of methanol were produced worldwide in 1991, principally by catalytic conversion of pressurized synthesis gas (hydrogen, carbon dioxide and carbon monoxide). Worldwide capacity was projected to rise to 30 million tonnes by 1995.

Methanol is used in the industrial production of many important organic compounds, principally methyl tertiary butyl ether (MTBE), formaldehyde, acetic acid, glycol methyl ethers, methylamine, methyl halides and methyl methacrylate.

Methanol is a constituent of a large number of commercially available solvents and consumer products including paints, shellacs, varnishes, paint thinners, cleansing solutions, antifreeze solutions, automotive windshield washer fluids and deicers, duplicating fluids, denaturant for ethanol, and in hobby and craft adhesives. Potentially large uses of methanol are in its direct use as a fuel, in gasoline blends or as a gasoline extender. It should be noted that the highest morbidity and mortality has been associated with deliberate or accidental oral ingestion of methanol-containing mixtures.

Methanol has been identified in exhausts from both gasoline and diesel engines and in tobacco smoke.

1.3   Environmental levels and human exposure

Emissions of methanol primarily occur from the miscellaneous industrial and domestic solvent use, methanol production, end-product manufacturing and bulk storage and handling losses.

Exposures to methanol can occur in occupational settings through inhalation or dermal contact. Many national occupational health exposure limits suggest that workers are protected from any adverse effects if exposures do not exceed a time-weighted average of 260 mg/m^3 (200 ppm) methanol for any 8-h day and for a 40-h working week.

Current general population exposures through air are typically 10 000 times lower than occupational limits. The general population is exposed to methanol in air at concentrations ranging from less than

0.001 mg/m^3 (0.8 ppb) in rural air to nearly 0.04 mg/m^3 (30 ppb) in urban air.

Data on the occurrence of methanol in finished drinking-water is limited, but methanol is frequently found in industrial effluents.

If the projected use of methanol as an alternate fuel or in admixture with fuels increases significantly, it can be expected that there will be widespread exposure to methanol via inhalation of vapours from methanol-fuelled vehicles and/or siphoning or percutaneous absorption of methanol fuels or blends.

1.4 Environmental distribution and transformation

Methanol is readily degraded in the environment by photo oxidation and biodegradation processes. Half-lives of 7-18 days have been reported for the atmospheric reaction of methanol with hydroxyl radicals.

Many genera and strains of microorganisms are capable of using methanol as a growth substrate. Methanol is readily degradable under both aerobic and anaerobic conditions in a wide variety of environmental media including fresh and salt water, sediments and soils, ground water, aquifer material and industrial wastewater; 70% of methanol in sewage systems is generally degraded within 5 days.

Methanol is a normal growth substrate for many soil microorganisms, which are capable of completely degrading methanol to carbon dioxide and water.

Methanol has a fairly low absorptive capacity on soils. Bioconcentration in most organisms is low.

Methanol is of low toxicity to aquatic and terrestrial organisms, and effects due to environmental exposure to methanol are unlikely to be observed except in the case of a spill.

1.5 Absorption, distribution, biotransformation and elimination

Methanol is readily absorbed by inhalation, ingestion and dermal exposure, and it is rapidly distributed to tissues according to the distribution of body water. A small amount of methanol is excreted unchanged by the lungs and kidneys.

Following ingestion, peak serum levels occur within 30-90 min, and methanol is distributed throughout the body with a volume of distribution of approximately 0.6 litre/kg.

Methanol is metabolized primarily in the liver by sequential oxidative steps to formaldehyde, formic acid and carbon dioxide. The initial step involves oxidation to formaldehyde by hepatic alcohol dehydrogenase, which is a saturable rate-limiting process. The relative affinity of alcohol dehydrogenase for ethanol and methanol is approximately 20:1. In step 2, formaldehyde is oxidized by formaldehyde dehydrogenase to formic acid/or formate depending on the pH. In step 3, formic acid is detoxified to carbon dioxide by folate-dependent reactions.

Elimination of methanol from the blood via the urine and exhaled air and by metabolism appears to be slow in all species, especially when compared to ethanol. Clearance proceeds with reported half-times of 24 h or more with doses greater than 1 g/kg and half-times of 2.5-3 h for doses less than 0.1 g/kg. It is the rate of metabolic detoxification, or removal of formate that is vastly different between rodents and primates and is the basis for the dramatic differences in methanol toxicity observed between rodents and primates.

1.6 Effects on laboratory mammals and *in vitro* test systems

1.6.1 Systemic toxicity

The acute and short-term toxicity of methanol varies greatly between different species, toxicity being highest in species with a relatively poor ability to metabolize formate. In such cases of poor metabolism of formate, fatal methanol poisoning occurs as a result of metabolic acidosis and neuronal toxicity, whereas, in animals that readily metabolize formate, consequences of CNS depression (coma, respiratory failure, etc.) are usually the cause of death. Sensitive primate species (humans and monkeys) develop increased blood formate concentrations following methanol exposure, while resistant rodents, rabbits and dogs do not. Humans and non-human primates are uniquely sensitive to the toxic effects of methanol. Overall methanol has a low acute toxicity to non-primate animals. The LD_{50} values and minimal lethal doses after oral exposure range from 7000 to 13 000 mg/kg in the rat, mouse, rabbit and dog and from 2000 to 7000 mg/kg for the monkey.

Rats exposed to levels of methanol up to 6500 mg/m^3 (5000 ppm) for 6 h/day, 5 days/week for 4 weeks, exhibited no exposure-related effects except for increased discharges around the nose and eyes. These were considered reflective of upper respiratory irritation.

Rats exposed to methanol vapour levels up to 13 000 mg/m^3 (10 000 ppm) for 6 h/day, 5 days/week for 6 weeks, failed to demonstrate pulmonary toxicity.

In the rabbit, methanol is a moderately irritant to the eye. It was not skin-sensitizing in a modified maximization test.

Toxic effects found in methanol-exposed primates include metabolic acidosis and ocular toxicity, effects that are not normally found in folate-sufficient rodents. The differences in toxicity are due to differences in the rate of metabolism of the methanol metabolite formate. For instance, the clearance of formate from the blood of exposed primates is at least 50% slower than for rodents.

Monkeys receiving methanol doses higher than 3000 mg/kg by gavage demonstrated ataxia, weakness and lethargy within a few hours of exposure. These signs tended to disappear within 24 h and were followed by transient coma in some of the animals.

In monkeys exposed to methanol for 6 h/day for 5 days a week, 20 repeated exposures to 6500 mg/m^3 (5000 ppm) methanol failed to elicit ocular effects.

1.6.2   Genotoxicity and carcinogenicity

Methanol has given negative results for gene mutation in bacteria and yeast assays, but it did induce chromosomal malsegregation in Aspergillus. It did not induce sister chromatic exchanges in Chinese hamster cells *in vitro* but caused significant increases in mutation frequencies in L5178Y mouse lymphoma cells.

Methanol inhalation did not induce chromosomal damage in mice. There is some evidence that oral or intraperitoneal administration increased the incidence of chromosomal damage in mice.

There is no evidence from animal studies to suggest that methanol is a carcinogen, although the lack of an appropriate animal model is recognized.

1.6.3   Reproductive toxicity, embryotoxicity and teratogenicity

Conflicting results have been reported on the effects of inhalation of methanol for up to six weeks on gonadotropin and testosterone concentrations.

The inhalation of methanol by pregnant rodents throughout the period of embryogenesis induces a wide range of concentration-dependent teratogenic and embryolethal effects. Treatment-related malformations, predominantly extra or rudimentary cervical ribs and urinary or cardiovascular defects, were found in fetuses of rats exposed 7 h/day for 7-15 days of gestation to 26 000 mg/m^3 (20 000 ppm) methanol. Slight maternal toxicity was found at this exposure level, and no adverse effects to the mother or offspring were found in animals exposed to 6500 mg/m^3 (5000 ppm), which was interpreted as the no-observed-adverse-effect level (NOAEL) for this test system.

Increased incidences of exencephaly and cleft palate were found in the offspring of CD-1 mice exposed 7 h/day, on days 6-15 of gestation, to methanol levels of 6500 mg/m^3 (5000 ppm) or more. There was increased embryo/fetal death at 9825 mg/m^3 (7500 ppm) or more and an increasing incidence of full-litter resorptions. Reduced fetal weight was observed at 13 000 and 19 500 mg/m^3 (10 000 or 15 000 ppm). The NOAEL for developmental toxicity was 1300 mg/m³ (1000 ppm) methanol. There was no evidence of maternal toxicity at methanol exposure levels below 9000 mg/m³ (7000 ppm).

When litters of pregnant CD-1 mice were given 4 g methanol/kg by gavage, the incidences of adverse effects on resorption, external defects including cleft palate, and fetal weight were similar to those found in the 13 000 mg/m³ (10 000 ppm) inhalation exposure group, presumably due to the greater rate of respiration of the mouse. The mouse is more sensitive than the rat to developmental toxicity resulting from inhaled methanol.

Transient neurological signs and reduced body weights were found in CD-1 dams exposed to 19 500 mg/m³ (15 000 ppm) for 6 h/day throughout organogenesis (gestational days 6-15). Fetal malformations found at 13 000 and 19 500 mg/m³ (10 000 and 15 000 ppm) included neural and ocular defects, cleft palate, hydronephrosis and limb anomalies.

1.7 Effects on humans

Humans (and non-human primates) are uniquely sensitive to methanol poisoning and the toxic effects in these species is characterized by formic acidaemia, metabolic acidosis, ocular toxicity, nervous system depression, blindness, coma and death. Nearly all of the available information on methanol toxicity in humans relates to the consequences of acute rather than chronic exposures. A vast majority of poisonings involving methanol have occurred from drinking adulterated beverages and from methanol-containing products. Although ingestion dominates as the most frequent route of poisoning, inhalation of high concentrations of methanol vapour and percutaneous absorption of methanolic liquids are as effective as the oral route in producing acute toxic effects. The most noted health consequence of longer-term exposure to lower levels of methanol is a broad range of ocular effects.

The toxic properties of methanol are based on factors that govern both the conversion of methanol to formic acid and the subsequent metabolism of formate to carbon dioxide in the folate pathway. The toxicity is manifest if formate generation continues at a rate that exceeds its rate of metabolism.

The lethal dose of methanol for humans is not known for certain. The minimum lethal dose of methanol in the absence of medical treatment is between 0.3 and 1 g/kg. The minimum dose causing permanent visual defects is unknown.

The severity of the metabolic acidosis is variable and may not correlate well with the amount of methanol ingested. The wide interindividual variability of the toxic dose is a prominent feature in acute methanol poisoning.

Two important determinants of human susceptibility to methanol toxicity appear to be (1) concurrent ingestion of ethanol, which slows the entrance of methanol into the metabolic pathway, and (2) hepatic folate status, which governs the rate of formate detoxification.

The symptoms and signs of methanol poisoning, which may not appear until after an asymptomatic period of about 12 to 24 h, include visual disturbances, nausea, abdominal and muscle pain, dizziness, weakness and disturbances of consciousness ranging from coma to clonic seizures. Visual disturbances generally develop between 12 and 48 h after methanol ingestion and range from mild photophobia and misty or blurred vision to markedly reduced visual acuity and complete blindness. In extreme cases death results. The principal clinical feature is severe metabolic acidosis of the anion-gap type. The acidosis is largely attributed to the formic acid produced when methanol is metabolized.

The normal blood concentration of methanol from endogenous sources is less than 0.5 mg/litre (0.02 mmol/litre), but dietary sources may increase blood methanol levels. Generally, CNS effects appear above blood methanol levels of 200 mg/litre (6 mmol/litre); ocular symptoms appear above 500 mg/litre (16 mmol/litre), and fatalities have occurred in untreated patients with initial methanol levels in the range of 1500-2000 mg/litre (47-62 mmol/litre).

Acute inhalation of methanol vapour concentrations below 260 mg/m^3 or ingestion of up to 20 mg methanol/kg by healthy or moderately folate-deficient humans should not result in formate accumulation above endogenous levels.

Visual disturbances of several types (blurring, constriction of the visible field, changes in colour perception, and temporary or permanent blindness) have been reported in workers who experienced methanol air levels of about 1500 mg/m^3 (1200 ppm) or more.

A widely used occupational exposure limit for methanol is 260 mg/m^3 (200 ppm), which is designed to protect workers from any of the effects of methanol-induced formic acid metabolic acidosis and ocular and nervous system toxicity.

No other adverse effects of methanol have been reported in humans except minor skin and eye irritation at exposures well above 260 mg/m^3 (200 ppm).

1.8   Effects on organisms in the environment

LC$_{50}$ values in aquatic organisms range from 1300 to 15 900 mg/litre for invertebrates (48-h and 96-h exposures), and 13 000 to 29 000 mg/litre for fish (96-h exposure).

Methanol is of low toxicity to aquatic organisms, and effects due to environmental exposure to methanol are unlikely to be observed, except in the case of a spill.

2. IDENTITY, PHYSICAL AND CHEMICAL PROPERTIES, ANALYTICAL METHODS

2.1 Identity

Chemical formula: CH_3OH

Chemical structure:

$$H-\overset{\displaystyle H}{\underset{\displaystyle H}{C}}-OH$$

Relative molecular mass: 32.04

CAS chemical name: methanol

CAS registry number: 67-56-1

RTECS number: PC 1400000

Synonyms: methyl alcohol, carbinol, wood alcohol, wood spirits, wood naphtha, Columbian spirits, Manhattan spirits, colonial spirit, hydroxymethane, methylol, methylhydroxide, monohydroxymethane, pyroxylic spirit

Impurities in commercial methanol include acetone, acetaldehyde, acetic acid and water.

2.2 Physical and chemical properties

2.2.1 Physical properties

Methanol is a colourless, volatile, flammable liquid with a mild alcoholic odour when pure. However, the crude product may have a repulsive pungent odour. Methanol is miscible with water, alcohols, esters, ketones and most other solvents and forms many azeotropic mixtures. It is only slightly soluble in fats and oils (Clayton & Clayton, 1982; Windholz, 1983; Elvers et al., 1990).

Important physical constants and properties of methanol are summarized in Table 1.

Table 1. Some physical properties of methanol[a]

Appearance	clear colourless liquid
Odour	slight alcoholic when pure; crude material pungent
Boiling point	64.7°C
Flash point	15.6°C (open cup) 12.2°C (closed cup)
Freezing point	-97.68°C
Specific gravity	0.7915 (20/4°C) 0.7866 (25°C)

Vapour pressure
    at 30 °C
    at 20 °C
	
	160 mmHg
	92 mmHg

Henry's Law Constant (25 °C)	1.35×10^{-4} atm.m^3/mole
Log P (octanol/water)	- 0.82; -0.77; -0.68
Partition constant	-0.66; -0.64
Ignition temperature	470 °C
Explosive limits in air (% by volume)	lower 5.5 upper 44
Refractive index n^{20}	1.3284

[a] Data from: Clayton & Clayton, 1982; Elvers et al.,1990; Grayson, 1981; Howard, 1990; Windholz, 1983.

In the USA, sales grade methanol must normally meet the following specifications:

methanol content (weight %) minimum	99.85
acetone and aldehydes (ppm) maximum	30
acid (as acetic acid) (ppm) maximum	30
water content (ppm) maximum	1.500
specific gravity (d_{20}^{20})	0.7928
permanganate time, minimum	30
odour	characteristic
distillation range at 101 kPa	1 °C, must include 64.6 °C
colour, platinum-cobalt scale, maximum	5
appearance	clear-colourless
residual on evaporation, g/100 ml	0.001
carbonizable impurities, colour	30
platinum-cobalt scale, maximum	5

Grade AA differs in specifying an acetone maximum (20 ppm), a minimum for ethanol (10 ppm), and in having a more stringent water content specification (1.000 ppm, maximum) (Grayson, 1981).

2.2.2   Chemical properties

Methanol undergoes reactions that are typical of alcohols as a chemical class. The reactions of particular industrial importance include the following: dehydrogenation and oxidative dehydrogenation over silver or molybdenum-iron oxide to form formaldehyde; the acid-catalysed reaction with isobutylene to form methyl tertiary butyl ether (MTBE); carbonylation to acetic acid catalysed by cobalt or rhodium;

esterification with organic acids and acid derivatives; etherification; addition to unsaturated bonds and replacement of the hydroxyl group (Grayson, 1981; Elvers et al., 1990).

2.3 Conversion factors

1 ppm = 1.31 mg/m^3 (25 °C, 1013hPa) 1 mmol/litre = 32 mg/litre

1 mg/m^3 = 0.763 ppm (25 °C, 1013hPa) 1 mg/litre =31.2 µmol/litre

(Adapted from Clayton & Clayton, 1982)

2.4 Analytical methods

Prior to the advent of sensitive gas chromatographic techniques, the analysis of methanol in environmental, consumer and biological samples was performed by procedures involving isolation of the volatile alcohol and titrimetry. This was followed later by more sensitive spectrophotometric methods based on the oxidation of methanol to formaldehyde with potassium permanganate then reaction with Schiff's reagent or rosaniline solution to produce an easily recognizable and stable colour (Gettler, 1920; Boos, 1948; Skaug, 1956; Hindberg & Wieth, 1963; NIOSH, 1976).

The earliest procedures for the determination of methanol in blood and urine were based on the initial distillation to isolate the volatile alcohol (Gettler, 1920). Feldstein & Klendshog (1954) determined methanol in biological fluids by initial microdiffusion followed by oxidation to formaldehyde and subsequent reaction with chromotropic acid (1,8-dihydroxy naphthalene-3,6-disulfonic acid). The recovery ranged from 80 to 85% for less than 0.10 mg methanol. In the procedure of Harger (1935), methanol was determined by oxidation with bichromate to carbon dioxide and water followed by titration with a mixture of ferrous sulfate and methyl orange. Jaselkis & Warriner (1966) determined methanol in aqueous solution by titrimetry employing xenon trioxide oxidation. Methanol was determined at a level of 0.03 mg with a relative standard deviation of 4%.

2.4.1 Environmental samples

The determination of methanol by primarily GC-FID procedures has been frequently reported in ambient air, workplace air, fuels, fuel emissions, sewage and aqueous solutions, soils, coal-gasification condensate water and tobacco smoke.

The measurement of methanol in ambient and workplace air, usually involves a preconcentration step in which the sample is passed through a solid absorbent containing silica gel, Tenax GC, Porapak or activated charcoal (NIOSH, 1976,1977,1984; CEC, 1988). It can also be accomplished by on-column cryogenic trapping or can be analysed directly. Direct reading infrared instruments with gas cuvettes can be used for continuous monitoring of methanol in air (Lundberg, 1985).

2.4.1.1 Methanol in air

The use of absorption tubes to trap methanol from ambient and workplace air with subsequent liquid or thermal desorption prior to gas chromatographic analysis has been reported frequently. The US National Institute of Occupational Safety and Health (NIOSH, 1977,1984) recommended the use of a glass tube (7 cm x 4 mm internal diameter) containing two sections of 20-40 mesh silica gel separated by a 2-mm portion of urethane foam (front=100 mg, back=50 mg). Water is used to extract the methanol, which is separated on a 2 m x 2 mm internal diameter glass column containing 60-80 mesh Tenax GC or the equivalent using flame ionization detection (FID). The working range is 25 to 900 mg/m^3 (19 to 690 ppm) methanol for a 5-litre air sample. The limit of detection has been reported to be 1.05 mg/m^3 in a 3-litre air sample (NIOSH, 1976). At high concentrations of methanol or at high relative humidity, a large silica gel tube is required (700 mg silica gel front section). The injection, detector and column temperatures are 200 °C, 250-300 °C and 80 °C respectively. Positive identification by mass spectrometry may be necessary in some cases, and alternative gas chromatographic columns, e.g., SP-1000, SP-2100 or FFAP, are also conformation aides.

Although GC-FID provides greater sensitivity than GC-MS, the latter is generally considered more reliable for the measurement of methanol in samples containing other alcohols or low molecular weight oxygenates.

Analysis of methanol in workplace air has been carried out by head-space GC-FID using a column containing 15% Carbowax 1500 on diatomaceous earth, 70-100 mesh operated at 100 °C. The detection limit was below 5 ml/m^3 (Heinrich & Angerer, 1982). Methanol in workplace air was initially collected in silica gel tubes and the methanol concentrations analysed by GC-FID equipped with a 50 m silica capillary column containing Carbowax 20M. Additionally, methanol vapour concentrations in the workplace have been analysed by a Miron-B analyser with detection at a wavelength of 9.70 μm.

Methanol and other low molecular weight oxygenates have been determined in ambient air by cryogradient sampling and two-dimensional gas chromatography (Jonsson & Berg, 1983). Samples were initially separated on a packed column (1,2,3-tris (2-cyanoethoxy)propane on Chromosorb W-AW), then refocused on-line in a fused-silica capillary cold trap, followed by on-line splitless reinjection onto a 50 m x 0.3 mm internal diameter fused silica capillary column. The detection limit for a typical oxygenate (3-methylbutanol) was 0.1 μg/m^3 using a 3-litre sample. The detection limit for methanol was slightly higher.

Spectrophotometric methods have also been employed for the determination of methanol in air. Aqueous potassium permanganate acidified with phosphoric acid was used to absorb methanol from air with the simultaneous oxidation to formaldehyde. After the addition of *p*-aminoazobenzene and sulfur dioxide, the resulting pink dye was determined spectrophotometrically at 505 nm. The limit of detection was 5 μg methanol/ml air (Verma & Gupta, 1984).

Methanol from air was absorbed by acidified potassium permanganate producing formaldehyde which on reaction with 4-nitroaniline produced a yellow dye determined spectroscopically at 395 nm (Upadhyay & Gupta, 1984).

Infrared spectrometry and infrared lasers have also been employed for the determination of methanol in air (Diaz-Rueda et al., 1977; Sweger & Travis, 1979). Methanol together with acetone, toluene and ethyl acetate were recovered from 10 litres of air at a flow rate of 11 ml/min by passage through a tube containing 150 mg of activated charcoal. The carbon disulfide extracts of the organic compounds were determined by infrared at 1300 cm^{-1} using caesium bromide windows. The minimum concentration of methanol detected quantitatively was 0.77 mg/m³ (0.60 ppm) and the minimum concentration required for identification was 0.24 mg/m³ (0.18 ppm) (Diaz-Rueda et al., 1977).

Infrared lasers have been used to detect trace organic gases including methanol. An air sample at 8 Tor was introduced to a 20-litre capacity sample cell, and laser radiation was detected synchronously by a mercury-cadmium Te detector. The laser line employed was P (34), the electric field was 1.40 kV/cm and the measurement time was 2 min. The detection limit for methanol was 0.105 mg/m³ (0.08 ppm) (Sweger & Travis, 1979).

Methanol in the workplace can be measured by portable direct reading instruments, real-time continuous monitoring systems and passive dosimeters (NIOSH, 1976,1977,1984; Liesivouri & Savolainen, 1987; Kawai et al., 1990).

Kawai et al. (1990) described a personal diffusive badge type that could absorb methanol vapour in linear relation to the exposure duration up to 10 h and to exposure concentrations up to 1050 mg/m³ (800 ppm) the maximum duration and concentration tested respectively. Additionally it was shown that the response to short-term peak exposure was rapid enough and that no spontaneous desorption would occur.

2.4.1.2   Methanol in fuels

Agarawal (1988) determined methanol quantitatively in commercial gasoline via an initial extraction with ethylene glycol then by GC utilizing a GB-1 fused silica capillary column (OV-1 equivalent, 60 m x 0.32 mm internal diameter) and FID. The recovery of 4% methanol in gasoline by this procedure was 95.4 ± 2.34% (SD).

In the procedure of Tackett (1987), gasoline samples were injected directly on a Carbowax 20M column operated at 50 °C for 3.0 min and then programmed to rise to 150 °C at a rate of 10 °C per min. The calibration curve is linear up to 10% (v/v) methanol and the detection limit was 0.2% employing a thermal conductivity detector.

Low molecular weight alcohols and MTBE were determined in gasoline by GC-FID utilizing dual columns: 4.6 m x 3.2 mm o.d. column packed with 30% m/m ethylene glycol succinate on

Chromosorb P (85-100 mesh) and a 2.7 m x 3.2 mm o.d. stainless steel column packed with Porapak P (80-100 mesh) operated at 150 °C (Luke & Ray, 1984).

Gas chromatographic analyses of methanol, ethanol and *tert*-butanol in gasoline have been reported by Pauls & McCoy (1981). The GC column was 150 cm x 3 mm in o.d. stainless steel packed with Porapak R (80-100 mesh) operated at 175 °C and the injector and FID detector temperatures were maintained at 250 °C.

A direct liquid chromatographic method for the determination of C1-C3 alcohols and water in gasoline-alcohol blends was described by Zinbo (1984). The separation was performed on either one or two microparticulate size-exclusion columns of ultrastyragel with toluene as the mobile phase. The quantification of alcohols and water in the effluent was achieved by a differential refractometer at 30 °C. The lower limits of detection for C1-C3 alcohols was 0.005 vol %. Methanol in gasoline-alcohol blends has been determined by nuclear magnetic resonance (Renzoni et al., 1985). The method takes advantage of a window in the proton nuclear magnetic resonance spectrum of gasoline that extends from a chemical shift of 2.8 to 6.8 ppm. Methanol was quantified in gasoline by integration of the methyl singlet at 3.4 ppm. The method gave linear calibration curves in the range of 0-25% (v/v) methanol with a detection limit of less than 0.1%.

4.1.3 Methanol in fuel emissions

Methanol has been detected in motor vehicle emissions at levels of 0.9 mg/m^3 (0.69 ppm) and in ambient air by GC-FID utilizing a 360 cm x 0.27 cm internal diameter stainless steel column packed with Porapak Q (50-80 mesh) operated at 150 °C (Bellar & Sigsby, 1970).

Seizinger & Dimitriades (1972) determined methanol in simple hydrocarbon fuel emissions utilizing GC with time-of-flight mass spectrometry. The analytical procedure involved concentration of the exhaust oxygenates drawn through a Chromosorb bed followed by GC-FID initially on a 30 in by 1/4 in o.d. column packed with 10% 1,2,3-tris (2-cyanoethoxy) propane (TCEP) programmed from -20 °C to 110 °C at 4 °C /min. The second-stage column was a 45 m x 0.05 cm internal diameter by 0.03 o.d Carbowax 20M support coated on tubular (SCOT) column programmed from 60 °C to 210 °C at

10 °C/min. The column effluent was split for parallel detection with FID and mass spectrometry. Methanol was found at levels of 0.1-0.8 mg/m^3 (0.1-0.6 ppm) in the exhaust of simple hydrocarbon fuels.

Methods for the quantification of evaporative emissions (running losses, hot soak, diurnal and refuelling) from methanol-fuelled motor vehicles (methanol/gasoline fuel mixtures of 100, 85, 50, 15 and 0% methanol) have been described (Snow et al., 1989; Federal Register, 1989; Gabele & Knapp, 1993).

Methanol emissions from methanol-fuelled cars were determined by GC employing a Quadrex 007 methyl silicone 50 m x 0.53 mm internal diameter column with 5.0 μm film thickness. The separation was affected isothermally at 75 °C (limit of detection 0.25 μg/ml) (Williams et al., 1990).

2.4.1.4 *Methanol in sewage and aqueous solutions*

Fox (1973) determined methanol at levels of 0.5-100 mg/litre (0.5-100 ppm) in sewage or other aqueous solutions by GC-FID employing a 0.5 m x 3.175 mm o.d. stainless steel column packed with Tenax GC 60/80 mesh and operated at 70 °C isothermal.

C_1-C_4 alcohols in aqueous solution were determined quantitatively by GC-FID using a 1 m x 0.32 cm stainless steel column packed with 5% w/w Carbowax 20M on Chromosorb 101 (80-100 mesh) with a column temperature of 65 °C for methanol and ethanol and 100 °C for *n*-propanol and *n*-butanol (Sims, 1976).

Methanol and ethanol at the mg/litre level in aqueous solution were determined by Komers & Sir (1976) utilizing a combination of stripping and GC-FID technique. The alcohols were analysed as their corresponding volatile nitrite on a 170 cm x 0.4 cm internal diameter glass column containing Chromosorb 102 (80-120 mesh) operated at 104 °C. Approximately 1 μg of the individual alcohol could be determined in sample volumes of about 5 ml.

Mohr & King (1985) determined methanol in coal-gasification condensate water by GC. Condensate water was injected directly on a 45 x 0.32 cm Porapak R column programmed from 80-200 °C at 20 °C/min.

A standard method for the analysis of methanol in raw, waste and potable waters has been published by the UK Standing Committee of Analysts (1982). The method is based on direct injection GC-FID using a 2 m stainless steel column with 15% carbowax 1540 m chromosorb W80-100 DMCS. The limit of detection is 0.11 mg/litre.

4.1.5   *Methanol in soils*

The biodegradation of methanol in gasolines by various soils was determined by Novak et al. (1985). Methanol extracted in water (25% v/v) was measured by direct injection GC-FID using a 2.1 m x 3 mm stainless steel column packed with 0.2% Carbowax 1500 0n 80/100 mesh Carbopak C at 120 °C isothermal.

2.4.2   **Foods, beverages and consumer products**

Lund et al. (1981) determined methanol in orange and grapefruit juice, fresh and canned, by GC-FID using a 1.5 x 3 mm column packed with 50/80 mesh Porapak Q at 100 °C with injector port and detector block at 200 °C.

Greizerstein (1981) utilized GC-FID and GC-MS for the analysis of alcohols, aldehydes and esters in commercial beverages (beers, wines, distilled spirits). Separations were carried out using a 3 m x 2 mm internal diameter glass column packed with 30% Carbowax 20 M at 150 °C. A more satisfactory separation of methanol from the other congeners was achieved using a 180-cm Porapak P column. Methanol was found at levels of 6-27 mg/litre beer; 96-321 mg/litre in wines and 10-220 mg/litre in distilled spirits. Methanol in distilled liquors and cordials has been determined by GC-FID (AOAC, 1990).

Rastogi (1993) analysed methanol content of 26 model and hobby glues and found methanol in 12 of them by head-space GC-FID employing capillary columns of different polarity. The polar GC column was a Supelcowax 10, 60 m x 0.32 mm internal diameter; and the non-polar column was a CP-Sil-5 CB, 50 m x 0.32 mm. The detection limit for methanol was 20 mg/litre.

Methanol in wine vinegars was determined by GC-MS (Blanch et al., 1992). Methanol with many other minor volatile components was fractionated using a simultaneous distillation extraction technique before GC analysis on a 4 m x 0.85 mm internal diameter micropacked column coated with a mixture of Carbowax and bis-(2-ethylhexyl)-sebecate (92:8), 4% on desilanized Volaspher A-2. The column temperature was 60 °C and the injector and FID detector were at 180 °C.

2.4.3   Biological materials

A variety of primarily gas chromatographic methods have been utilized for the determination of methanol in biological samples from normal, poisoned and occupationally exposed individuals. Methanol exposure has been measured in exhaled breath, blood and urine samples.

2.4.3.1   Methanol in exhaled air

Prior to analysis, expired air samples are normally collected in sampling bags or glass containers or after preconcentration on Tenax or other solid sorbents in adsorbent tubes and thermally desorbed, or utilizing cryotraps (Franzblau et al., 1992a).

Free methanol has been detected and measured by GC in the expired air of normal healthy humans with separations made on 1.52 m x 0.3 cm columns filled with Anakrom ABS, 70-80 mesh coated with 2% N,N,-N,-N-tetramethyl azeleamide and 8% behenyl alcohol at 86 °C. The concentration of methanol in nine subjects ranged from 0.06-0.32 µg/litre (Eriksen & Kulkarni, 1963). Methanol was only infrequently detected in samples of human expired air and saliva by Larsson (1965) employing GC-FID and a 1.75 mx 3.5 mm internal diameter glass column containing polyethylene glycol (M=1500) 20% on Chromosorb W.

Methanol in expired air and in head-space analysis of plasma was determined as the nitrite ester utilizing GC-MS (Jones et al., 1983). Condensed expired air samples were analysed on Porapak Q and the assay of methanol nitrite ester was accomplished on a 2 m x 2 mm internal diameter silanized glass column containing Tenax GC (30-60 mesh) at 60 °C.

Krotosynski et al. (1977) analysed expired air from normal healthy subjects using for sample preconcentration a 18 cm x 6 mm o.d. stainless steel column containing Tenax GC. Sample analysis was performed using GC-FID and a 91 m x 6 mm stainless steel column coated with Emulphoron-870. Apart from methanol, 102 organic compounds were detected.

Alveolar air of workers exposed to methanol was first collected in gas sampling tubes and then analysed by GC-FID using a Porapak Q (80-100 mesh) column at 150 °C (Baumann & Angerer, 1979).

The detection of methanol and other endogenous compounds in expired air by GC-FID with on-column concentration of sample and separation on a 1.5 m x 3 mm o.d. stainless steel column packed with Porapak Q, 80-100 mesh maintained at 35 °C was described by Phillips & Greenberg (1987).

The expired air of volunteer subjects exposed for periods of about 90 min to atmospheres artificially contaminated with low levels of methanol (ca. 130 mg/m^3 (100 ppm)) was monitored during and after the exposure using an atmospheric pressure ionization mass spectrometer (API/MS) fitted with a direct breath analysis system (Benoit et al., 1985).

A transportable Fourier Transform Infrared (FTIR) spectrometer was utilized for the analysis of methanol vapour in alveolar and ambient air in humans exposed to methanol vapour. The infrared spectrum region used for methanol quantification was in the 950-1100 cm region. For the analysis of methanol in alveolar air with FTIR the limit of detection for methanol was 0.4 mg/m^3 (0.32 ppm), and for methanol in ambient air the detection limit was 0.13 mg/m^3 (0.1 ppm) (Franzblau et al., 1992a).

4.3.2 Methanol in blood

A number of methods have been used to extract methanol from blood prior to analysis including purge-and-trap, head-space analysis and solvent extraction.

Baker et al. (1969) reported the simultaneous determination of lower alcohols, acetone and acetaldehyde in blood by GC-FID utilizing a 183 cm x 5 mm internal diameter column containing Porapak Q operated at 100 °C. The method did not require precipitation of protein prior to analysis.

Methanol in whole blood and serum was analysed by GC-FID employing 1.2 m and 1.8 m x 3 mm internal diameter glass columns packed with 20% Hallcomid or 10% Carbowax on 60-80 mesh Diatopor TW operated at 70 °C (Mather & Assimos, 1965).

Blood serum was deproteinized and acetone and aliphatic alcohols including methanol were determined by GC-FID using a pre-column of 3% OV-1 on Gas Chrom Q and an analytical 30-m capillary column packed with SPB-1 and operated at 35 °C. Methanol and other alcohols were separated in less than 3 min (Smith, 1984).

Methanol in deproteinized blood samples from occupationally exposed workers was quantified by GC-FID employing a 1.8 m x 4 mm internal diameter glass column packed with 60-80 mesh Carbopak B/5% Carbowax 20M at 60 °C. The detection limit for methanol was about 0.4 µg/ml (Lee et al., 1992).

Methanol in blood of occupationally exposed workers was determined by head-space GC-FID utilizing a column containing 15% Carbowax 1599 on diatomaceous earth, 70-80 mesh and operated at 70 °C. The detection limit was 0.6 mg/litre (Heinrich & Angerer, 1982).

The simultaneous determination of methanol, ethanol, acetone, isopropanol and ethylene glycol in plasma by GC-FID was accomplished using a 180 cm x 4 mm internal diameter glass column packed with Porapak Q, 50-80 mesh. The column temperature was programmed from 199-210 °C at 2 °C/min, and the injection port and detector temperatures were 210 °C and 240 °C respectively. The detection limit for methanol was 0.1 nmol/ml. The procedure was recommended for methanol and ethylene glycol intoxication cases (Cheung & Lin, 1987).

Methanol in blood from occupationally exposed workers was determined directly without further pretreatment by GC-FID using a 4 m x 3 mm glass column packed with 10% SBS 100 on Shimalite TPA, 60-80 mesh. The detector and oven were heated at 180 °C and 60 °C, respectively (Kawai et al., 1991a).

Head-space GC-FID on methanol in blood from workers exposed at sub-occupational exposure limits was reported by Kawai et al. (1992). A 30 m x 0.53 mm capillary column coated with 1.0 um DB-

Wax was used with the injection port and detector heated at 200 °C and the oven temperature kept at 40 °C for 1 min after the injection and then elevated at a rate of 5 °C/min to 110 °C for 15 min. The detection limit for methanol in blood was 100 µg/litre.

Leaf & Zatman (1952) utilized a colorimetric procedure for the determination of methanol in air as well as in the blood and urine of occupationally exposed workers in a methanol synthesis plant. The procedure involved acid permanganate oxidation of methanol to formaldehyde, which was then determined with a modified Schiff's reagent. Concentrations of methanol up to 150 mg/litre were determined to within 3%.

Determination of methanol in patients with acute methanol poisoning was accomplished with a colorimetric procedure following permanganate oxidation to formaldehyde and the subsequent reaction with chromotropic acid (1,8-dihydroxy naphthalene 3,6-disulfonic acid). Quantitative recovery of 100% was found for methanol following the analysis of 3 ml of plasma, which required 45 min (Hindberg & Wieth, 1963).

Accumulation of methanol in blood was detected in alcoholic subjects during a 10-15 day period of chronic alcohol intake using GC-FID and a 1.8 m column packed with Porapak Q, 80-100 mesh, or Chromosorb 101 operated at 140 °C (Majchrowicz & Mendelson, 1971). The identity of methanol was also confirmed chemically using the specificity of the colour reaction between permanganate and formaldehyde.

Head-space GC was used to determine the concentrations of methanol and ethanol in blood samples from 519 individuals suspected of drinking and driving in Sweden. Methanol was determined in whole blood without prior dilution with an internal standard. Carbopack C (0.2% Carbowax 1500) was used as the stationary phase and the oven temperature was 80 °C (Jones & Lowinger, 1988).

Methanol in whole blood of poisoned patients was determined without pretreatment by GC-FID using a 1800 mm x 4 mm internal diameter glass column packed with 80-100 mesh Carbopack C/0.2% CW 1500 operated at 80 °C; the detector temperature was 120 °C (Jacobsen et al., 1982a).

Serum methanol concentrations in men after oral administration of the sweetening agent aspartame were determined by GC-MS utilizing a fused silica capillary column 26 m x 0.22 mm internal diameter of CPWAX 57 CB operated at 50 ° C isothermally (Davoli et al., 1986).

Methanol and formate in blood and urine of rats administered methanol intravenously was determined by HPLC employing a REZEX-ROA-organic acid column (300 mm x 7.8 mm internal diameter) and a similarly packed pre-column (50 mm x 4.6 mm internal diameter). The mobile phase was 0.043 N sulfuric acid with 10% acetonitrile at a flow rate of 1 ml/min (Horton et al., 1992).

Methanol in serum has also been determined by high-field (500 MHZ) proton nuclear magnetic resonance at the 3.39 singlet peak. For serum containing 20-500 mg of added methanol/litre, peak area was a linear function of concentration (r=0.998). This NMR technique permitted the determination of methanol and acetone in blood serum at a level of less than 1mM (Bock, 1982).

Pollack & Kawagoe (1991) determined methanol in deproteinized whole blood of rats by capillary GC-FID with direct column injection utilizing a 15 m x 0.54 mm internal diameter fused silica capillary column coated with Carbowax and operated at 35 °C. The limit of detection was 2 µg/ml.

2.4.3.3 Methanol in urine

Sedivec et al. (1981) determined methanol in urine in five volunteers exposed to methanol vapour for 8 h. Head-space GC-FID was used with a 120 cm x 3 mm column packed with Chromosorb 102, 60-80 mesh at 120 °C. The detection limit of methanol was 0.1 mg/litre. The methanol content in urine of 20 subjects occupationally exposed to methanol was determined by head-space GC-FID utilizing a column containing Porapak QS, 80-100 mesh and operated at 130 °C. The detection limit was 0.6 mg/litre (Heinrich & Angerer, 1982).

Methanol in the urine of exposed workers was determined by head-space GC-FID using a 4.1 m x 3.2 mm glass column containing 10% SBS-100 on Shimalite TPA, 60-80 mesh. The oven and injection port temperatures were 60 °C and 180 °C respectively. The limit of detection for methanol in urine was 0.1 mg/litre (Kawai et al., 1991b, 1992).

Urinary methanol as a measure of occupational exposure was determined by GC-FID utilizing a 2 m glass column packed with Porapak Q, 80-100 mesh. The detection limit for methanol was 0.32 mg/litre (Liesivouri & Savolainen, 1987).

Urine concentrations of methanol in volunteers who had ingested small amounts of methanol was determined by head-space GC-FID using Tenax GC as the column packing (Ferry et al., 1980).

4.3.4   *Methanol in miscellaneous biological tissues*

Methanol and other alcohols have been determined in tissue homogenates either *per se* or as their nitrite esters by GC-FID employing a 1.8 m x 6 mm o.d. glass column packed with Chromosorb 101 operated at 145 °C. The sensitivity was 8 µg per g of tissue (Gessner, 1970).

4.3.5   *Methanol metabolites in biological fluids*

The principal metabolite of methanol in humans and monkeys is formate and it has been shown that accumulation of blood formate at higher levels of methanol exposure coincides with the development of metabolic acidosis and visual system toxicities (Clay et al., 1975; McMartin et al., 1975; Baumbach et al., 1977; Tephly, 1991). Formate is an endogenous product of single carbon metabolism and is normally found in the urine of healthy individuals.

Formate has been analysed in blood and urine samples primarily by enzymatic methods with a colorimetric or fluorimetric end-point or by derivatization followed by analysis by GC-FID. Formate in plasma has also been determined by isotachophoresis (Sejersted et al., 1983).

Ferry et al. (1980) measured formic acid as an ethyl ester formed by the treatment of urine with 30% sulfuric acid in ethanol. The samples were analysed by head-space GC-FID on a column packed with 10% silar 10C on Chrom Q.

The analysis of formic acid in blood was performed via an initial transformation of formic acid by concentrated sulfuric acid into water and carbon monoxide, the latter being reduced to methane on a catalytic column and analysed directly by GC-FID (Angerer & Lehnert, 1977; Baumann & Angerer, 1979; Heinrich & Angerer, 1982).

Urinary formic acid was determined after the methylation of the acid and its conversion to N,N-dimethylformamide with GC-FID equipped with a 50-m silica capillary column containing Carbowax 20M liquid phase. The detection limit was 2.3 mg/litre (Liesivouri & Savolainen, 1987).

Franzblau et al. (1992b) found that urinary formic acid in specimens collected 16 h following cessation of methanol exposure and analysed by head-space GC-FID may not be an appropriate approach to assess methanol exposure biologically.

Enzymatic methods for the determination of formate are based primarily on the enzyme-catalysed conversion of formate to carbon dioxide in the presence of nicotinamide adenine dinucleotide (NAD), generating NADH as the other reaction product. NADH formation can be subsequently measured directly or reacted in a coupled reaction to generate a fluorescent or coloured complex.

A specific assay for formic acid in body fluids based on the reaction of formate with bacterial formate dehydrogenase coupled to a diaphorase-catalysed reduction of the non-fluorescent dye resazurin to the fluorescent substance resorufin was reported by Makar et al. (1975) and Makar & Tephly (1982). This permitted the accurate determination of about 6 mg formate/litre blood at excitation wavelength of 565 nm and an emission wavelength of 590 nm (Makar et al., 1975; Makar & Tephly, 1982).

A serum formate enzymic assay based on modifications of the formate dehydrogenase (FDH)-diaphorase procedure using NAD-diaphorase-iodonitrotetrazolium violet to develop a red-coloured complex, which is measured at 500 nm, was described by Grady & Osterloh (1986). The calibration curve was linear over the formate range of 0 to 400 mg/litre.

Formate in plasma was determined by Lee et al. (1992) employing an enzymatic procedure (Grady & Osterloh, 1986; Buttery

& Chamberlin, 1988) and measured spectrophotometrically at 510 nm. The detection limit was about 3 µg/ml.

Lee et al. (1992) determined that formate associated with acute methanol toxicity in humans does not accumulate in blood when atmospheric methanol exposure concentrations are below the occupational threshold limit value of 260 mg/m^3 (200 ppm) for 6 h in exposed healthy volunteers.

d'Alessandro et al. (1994) found that serum and urine formate determinations were not sensitive biological markers of methanol exposure at the threshold limit value (TLV) in human volunteers. Formate in serum was analysed by the enzymatic-colorimetric procedure of Grady & Osterloh (1986). The sensitivity of the method was 0.5 mg/litre of formate in serum.

Buttery & Chamberlin (1988) developed an enzymatic method for the determination of abnormal levels of formate in plasma requiring no deproteinization and utilizing a stable colour reagent consisting of phenazine methosulfate, *p*-iodonitrotetrazolium and NAD to produce a stable red formazan colour. The precision at 1.0 and 5.0 mmol/litre formate was 2.9% and 1.7%, respectively, within-day and 5.5% and 2.3%, respectively, between days.

Urinary formic acid was determined using formate dehydro-genase (FDH) in the presence of NAD. The detection limit was 0.5 mg/litre. The normal formic acid excretion in urine is between 2.0 and 30 mg/litre (Triebig & Schaller, 1980).

3. SOURCES OF HUMAN AND ENVIRONMENTAL EXPOSURE

3.1 Natural occurrence

Methanol occurs naturally in humans, animals and plants (Axelrod & Daly, 1965; CEC, 1988). It is a natural constituent of blood, urine and saliva (Leaf & Zatman, 1952) and expired air (Erikssen & Kulkarni, 1963; Larsson, 1965; Krotosynski et al., 1979; Jones et al., 1990), and has also been found in mother's milk (Pellizzari et al., 1982). Humans have a background body burden of 0.5 mg/kg body weight (Kavet & Nauss, 1990).

Levels of methanol in expired air are reported to range from 0.06 to 0.49 µg/litre (46-377 ppb) (Eriksen & Kulkarni, 1963). Methanol has been detected in the expired air of normal, healthy non-smoking subjects at a mean level of 0.5 ng/litre (Krotosynski et al., 1979).

It is believed that dietary sources are only partial contributors to the total body pool of methanol (Stegink et al., 1981). It has been suggested that methanol is formed by the activities of the intestinal microflora or by other enzymatic processes (Axelrod & Daly, 1965). The methanol-forming enzyme was shown to be protein carboxyl-methylase, an enzyme that methylates the carboxyl groups of proteins (Kim, 1973; Morin & Liss, 1973).

Natural emission sources of methanol include volcanic gasses, vegetation, microbes and insects (Owens et al., 1969; Holzer et al., 1977; Graedel et al., 1986). Isidorov et al. (1985) identified methanol emissions of evergreen cyprus in the forests of Northern Europe and Asia. Methanol was identified as one of the volatile components emitted by alfalfa (Owens et al., 1969) and it is formed during biological decomposition of biological wastes, sewage and sludges (US EPA, 1975; Howard, 1990; Nielsen et al., 1993).

3.2 Anthropogenic sources

The major anthropogenic sources of methanol include its production, storage and use, principally its use as a solvent, as a chemical intermediate, in the production of glycol ethers, and in the manufacture of charcoal, and exhaust from vehicle engines (US EPA, 1976a,b, 1980a,b; CEC, 1988).

3.2.1 Production levels and processes

.2.1.1 Production processes

The earliest important source of methanol ("wood alcohol") was the dry distillation of wood at about 350 °C, which was employed from around 1830 to 1930. In countries where wood is plentiful and wood products form an important industry, methanol is still obtained by this procedure (ILO, 1983).

In 1880, about 1.5 million litres of wood alcohol were produced in the USA while in 1910 the amount had increased to over 3 million litres (Tyson & Schoenberg, 1914). However methanol produced from wood contained more contaminants, primarily acetone, acetic acid and allyl alcohol, than the chemical-grade methanol currently available (Grayson, 1981; Elvers et al., 1990). Methanol was also produced as one of the products of the non-catalytic oxidation of hydrocarbons (a procedure discontinued in the USA in 1973), and as a by-product of Fischer-Tropsch synthesis, which is no longer industrially important (Grayson, 1981).

Modern industrial scale methanol production is based exclusively on the catalytic conversion of pressurized synthesis gas (hydrogen, carbon monoxide and carbon dioxide) in the presence of metallic heterogenous catalysts. All carbonaceous materials such as coal, coke, natural gas, petroleum and fractions obtained from petroleum (asphalt, gasoline, gaseous compounds) can be employed as starting materials for synthesis gas production (Grayson, 1981; Elvers et al., 1990).

The required synthesis pressure is dependant upon the activity of the particular metallic catalyst employed, with copper-containing zinc oxide-alumina catalysts being the most effective in industrial methanol plants (Elvers et al., 1990). By convention the processes are classified according to the pressure used: low-pressure processes, 50-100 atmospheres; medium-pressure processes, 100-250 atmospheres; and high-pressure processes, 250-350 atmospheres. Low-pressure technology is the most widely employed globally and accounted for 55% of the USA methanol capacity in 1980 (Grayson, 1981).

Almost all the methanol produced in the USA is made from natural gas. This is steam reformed to produce synthesis gas, which is converted to methanol by low-pressure processes. A small amount of methanol is obtained as a by-product from the oxidation of butane to produce acetic acid and from the destructive distillation of wood to produce charcoal (Grayson, 1981; Elvers et al., 1990).

The composition of methanol obtained directly from synthesis without any purification or with only partial purification varies according to the synthesis (e.g., pressure, catalyst, feedstock). The principal impurities include 5-20% (by volume) water, higher alcohols (principally ethanol), methyl formate and higher esters, and smaller amounts of ethers and aldehydes (Grayson, 1981; Elvers et al., 1990). Methanol is purified by distillation, the complexity required depending on the desired methanol purity and the purity of the crude methanol (Grayson, 1981; Elvers et al., 1990).

Natural gas, petroleum residues and naphtha accounted for 90% of worldwide methanol capacity in 1980, miscellaneous off-gas sources constituting the remaining 10%. Natural gas alone accounted for 70%, petroleum residues 15%, and naphtha 5% (Grayson, 1981). Natural gas feedstock accounted for 75% in the USA and 70% of global capacity in 1980. Methanol produced from residual oil accounted for approximately 15% of USA and worldwide capacity in 1980, while naphtha and coal feedstocks accounted for approximately 5% and 2%, respectively, of worldwide methanol capacity in 1980 (Grayson, 1981). About 90% of the global methanol capacity is currently based on natural gas (SRI, 1992).

The production of methanol from coal, being independent of oil and natural gas supplies, is noted to be an attractive alternative feed stock in some quarters (Grayson, 1981; CEC, 1988). Newer approaches to the production of methanol that have been suggested include the catalytic conversion from carbon dioxide and hydrogen avoiding conventional steam reforming (Rotman, 1994a) and the direct catalytic conversion of methane to methanol (Rotman, 1994b).

3.2.1.2 Production figures

As shown in Table 2, worldwide annual capacity for methanol production has increased over the past decades from approximately 15×10^6 tonnes in 1979 (Grayson, 1981) to 21×10^6 tonnes in 1989

Table 2. Methanol production or production capacity ($\times 10^6$ tonnes per year) from 1978 to 1995

Year	World-wide	USA	Canada	Western Europe	Japan	Capacity/production	Reference
1978	12	3.4		3	1	capacity production	Grayson (1981)
1979	15	4.05		3.45	1.35	capacity	Grayson (1981)
1980				2.5		production	CEC (1988)
1981	8					production	CEC (1988)
1983	15.9	5.52 (33%)	1.75 (11%)	2.53	1.27 (8%)	capacity production	SRI (1992) CEC (1988)
1988			1.91			production	Anderson (1993)
1989	21 19					capacity production	Elvers et al. (1990)
1990	22.3					capacity	Anon. (1991); Nielsen et al. (1993)
1991	22.1	4.42 (20%)	2.21 (10%)	2.65 (12%)[a]	0.22 (1%)	capacity	SRI (1992)
1991			2.22		0.077	production	Anderson (1993)
1992			2.15		0.034	production	Anderson (1993)
1992		3.66	2.15			production	Reisch (1994)
1993		4.78				production	Reisch (1994)
1995	30.1					capacity	SRI (1992)

[a] Only Germany, the Netherlands and the United Kingdom.

(Elvers et al., 1990) and more than 22.1 x 10^6 tonnes in the beginning of 1991 (SRI, 1992). Worldwide demand was projected to rise further to about 25.8 x 10^6 tonnes in 1994 (Anon., 1991; Nielsen et al., 1993) and 30.1 x 10^6 tonnes in 1995 (SRI, 1992). The data available do not allow capacity and production figures to be compared; however, it is assumed that approximately 80% of production capacity is utilized (Fiedler et al., 1990).

The USA and Canada are the largest methanol-producing countries. About 85% of Canada's production is exported to the USA, Japan and Europe (Heath, 1991). In Western Europe, Germany, the Netherlands and the United Kingdom are the major methanol-producing countries, accounting for 7%, 3% and over 2% of the world capacity, respectively (SRI, 1992). The production of methanol in Germany in 1991 and 1992 amounted to 715 000 and 770 000 tonnes respectively.

The annual capacity in Eastern Europe was estimated to be 5.8 x 10^6 tonnes in 1987. The production in the former USSR was 3.28 x 10^6 tonnes and 3.21 x 10^6 tonnes in 1987 and 1988, respectively (Rippen, 1990).

The figures in Table 2 indicate a major shift in methanol production from the developed countries to the developing areas. In fact, the methanol industry underwent large structural changes during the 1980s as a result of the discovery of large natural gas fields in remote regions having little demand for natural gas themselves. Since methanol production is a very suitable alternative for marketing natural gases, a number of methanol production plants for export were built or proposed to be built in Asia (Bahrein, Oman, Qatar, Saudi Arabia, Indonesia, Malaysia), South America (Chile, Mexico, Venezuela), the Caribbean (Trinidad) and in New Zealand and Norway (Fiedler et al., 1990; SRI, 1992). The largest single train plant based on this concept came on stream in southern Chile in 1988 with an annual output of 750 000 tonnes (Fiedler et al., 1990).

Future trends in methanol production and demand are being driven to a large extent by increasing demand for methyl tertiary butyl ether (MTBE), which is used in gasoline blending as an octane enhancer and to reduce carbon monoxide emissions (Anon., 1991; Morris, 1993; Nielsen et al., 1993).

3.2.2 *Uses*

During the 1890s, the market for methanol (then better known as wood alcohol) increased as a commercial product and as a solvent for use in the workplace. It was included in many consumer products such as witch hazel, Jamaica ginger, vanilla extract and perfumes (Wood & Buller, 1904). The most notorious use of wood alcohol was and continues to be as an adulterant in alcoholic beverages, which has led to large-scale episodes of poisonings since 1900 (Bennett et al., 1953; Kane et al., 1968).

Historically, in terms of commercial usage, about half of all methanol produced has been used to produce formaldehyde. Other earlier large-volume chemicals based on methanol include acetic acid, dimethyl terephthalate, glycol methyl ethers, methyl halides, methylamines, methyl acrylate and various solvent uses (Grayson, 1981; CEC, 1988; Elvers et al., 1990; Nielsen et al., 1993).

.2.2.1 *Use as feedstock for chemical syntheses*

Approximately 70% of the methanol produced worldwide is used as feedstock for chemical syntheses. As shown in Table 3, formaldehyde, methyl tertiary butyl ether (MTBE), acetic acid, methyl methacrylate, and dimethyl terephthalate are, in order of importance, the main chemicals produced from methanol. Methyl halides produced from methanol include methyl chloride, methylene chloride and chloroform.

Nearly all the formaldehyde manufactured worldwide is produced by oxidation of methanol with atmospheric oxygen. The annual formaldehyde production was projected to increase at a rate of 3%, but because other bulk products have higher growth rates, its relative importance with respect to methanol use has decreased (Elvers et al., 1990; Fiedler et al., 1990).

MTBE has become an important octane-enhancing blending component in gasoline, particularly in the USA where the Clean Air Act Amendments of 1990 have prompted further steps toward reducing emissions from motor vehicles by changing the formulations of gasoline. This is achieved by using so-called oxygenated fuel, i.e. fuel containing at least 2% oxygen by weight in the form of

Table 3. Use pattern for methanol (as a percentage of production) according to region and year

	Global	Global	USA	USA	Japan	Western Europe	Brazil
	1979	1988	1973	1985	n.g.	1985	n.g.
Use for synthesis of:							
formaldehyde	52	40	39	30	47	50	60
MTBE	4	20		8	-	5	-
acetic acid	6	9	3.4	12	10	5	-
dimethyl terephthalate	4		6.1	4	1	4	16
methyl methacrylate	4		3.7	4	6	3	2
methyl halides	8[a]		6.1	9	3	6	-
methyl amines			3.3	4	2	4	9
glycol methyl ethers			1.1				
Direct use							
solvent				10	6	6	2
fuel				6	-	5	-
Miscellaneous	14		16.9	13	25	12	11
Reference[b]	[1]	[2]	[3]	[4]	[4]	[4]	[4]

[a] together with methyl amines production
[b] Reference: [1] Kennedy & Shanks (1981); [2] Elvers et al. (1990); [3] US EPA (1980a); [4] Rippen (1990)
n.g. = year not given

oxygenates, but less benzene and other aromatic compounds than conventional fuel (Health Effects Institute, 1996). MTBE is produced by reacting methanol with isobutene in acid ion exchangers. In 1987, MTBE (production of 1.6×10^6 tonnes) ranked 32nd among the top 50 chemicals produced in the USA (Scholz et al., 1990). In 1993, 11×10^6 tonnes were produced, ranking MTBE ninth of the top 50 chemicals (Reisch, 1994).

Acetic acid is produced by carbonylation of methanol with carbon monoxide. Annual growth rates of 6% have been estimated (Fiedler et al., 1990).

Methanol is present in a broad variety of commercial and consumer products including shellacs, paints, varnishes, mixed solvents in duplicating machines (95% concentration or greater), antifreeze and gasoline deicers (generally containing 35-95% methanol), windshield washer fluid (contains 35-90% methanol), cleansing solutions (containing around 5% methanol), model and hobby glues and adhesives, and Sterno ("canned heat") containing 4% methanol (Posner, 1975; US EPA, 1980a; CEC, 1988; ATSDR, 1993).

Methanol is also used in the denitrification of wastewater, sewage treatment application (carbon source for bacteria to aid in the anaerobic conversion of nitrates to nitrogen and carbon dioxide), as a substrate for fermentation production of animal feed protein (single cell protein), as a hydrate inhibitor in natural gas, and in the methanolysis of polyethylene terephthalate (PET) from recycled plastic wastes (Posner, 1975; US EPA, 1980a; Kennedy & Shanks, 1981; ATSDR, 1993).

2.2.2   Use as fuel

Methanol is a potential substitute for petroleum. It can be directly used in fuel as a replacement for gasoline in gasoline and diesel blends. Methanol is in favour over conventional fuels because of its lower ozone-forming potential, lower emissions of some pollutants, particularly benzene and polycyclic aromatic hydrocarbons and sulfur compounds, and low evaporative emissions. On the other hand, the possibility of higher formaldehyde emissions, its higher acute toxicity and, at present, lower cost-efficiency favour conventional fuels (CONCAWE, 1995).

For use in gasoline engines, pure methanol (so-called M100 fuel) or mixtures of 3, 15 and 85% methanol with conventional petroleum products (M3, M15, M85) are most common. In diesel engines methanol cannot be used as an exclusive fuel because of its low cetane number that would impose proper ignition. Therefore, methanol is injected into the cylinder after ignition of the conventional diesel fuel (Fiedler et al., 1990).

3.2.2.3 Other uses

Methanol is used in refrigeration systems, e.g., in ethylene plants, and as an antifreeze in heating and cooling circuits. However, its use as an engine antifreeze has been replaced by glycol-based products. Methanol is added to natural gas at the pumping stations of pipelines to prevent formation of gas hydrates at low temperature and can be recycled after removal of water. Methanol is also used as an absorption agent in gas scrubbers to remove, for example, carbon dioxide and hydrogen sulfide. According to Table 3, large amounts of methanol are used as a solvent. Pure methanol is not usually used alone as a solvent, but is included in solvent mixtures (Fiedler et al., 1990).

3.2.2.4 Losses into the environment

Given the high production volume, widespread use and physical and chemical properties of methanol, there is a very high potential for large amounts of methanol to be released to the environment, principally to air (US EPA, 1976a,b, 1980a,b, 1994; Nielsen et al., 1993). Emissions of methanol primarily occur from miscellaneous solvent usage, methanol production, end-product manufacturing, and bulk storage and handling losses. The largest source of emissions of methanol is the miscellaneous solvent use category.

US EPA (1980b) estimated emission factors for the release of methanol and volatile organic compounds (VOC) from the low-pressure synthesis of methanol from natural gas in a model plant with a capacity of 450 000 tonnes/year. The process and capacity were typical of those built in the late 1970s. The overall emission factors were estimated to be: uncontrolled emissions, 1.56 kg methanol/tonne produced; controlled emissions, 0.14 kg methanol/tonne produced (Nielsen et al., 1993).

It was estimated that about 1% of the methanol used in the production of formaldehyde would be released to the environment during the production process by which formaldehyde is produced by either a metallic silver-catalyst process or a metal oxide-catalyst process (US EPA, 1976a; 1980b). In the oxidation-dehydrogenation process with metallic silver catalyst, 0.89 kg methanol/tonne of 39% (by weight) formaldehyde solution was released principally from the product absorber vents, and 1.24 kg methanol/tonne from the fractionator vents. The production of formaldehyde using the catalytic oxidation, metal oxide catalyst process resulted in the release of 1.93 kg methanol/tonne of 37% formaldehyde solution with emissions from the absorber vent (US EPA, 1980b).

US EPA (1994) reported that methanol was the most released chemical to the environment (air, water and land) based on the 1992 Toxic Release Inventory which utilized 81 016 individual chemical reports from a total of 23 630 facilities (approximately 65% of facilities reporting). The air, water and land releases of methanol totalled 1.09×10^5 tonnes, consisting of 1.53×10^4 tonnes of fugitive or non-point air emissions, 72 956 tonnes of stack or point air emissions, 7444 tonnes of surface water discharges and 15 095 tonnes released to land. Additionally, 1.283×10^4 tonnes were transferred via underground injection.

Methanol had the largest off-site transfers (51 672 tonnes) to publicly owned treatment works (POTWs) in 1992. During the same period, methanol ranked third largest of the Toxic Release Inventory Chemicals with off-site transfers for treatment. The total transfers to treatment were 18 098 tonnes, consisting of 4 tonnes for solidification, 10 295 tonnes for incineration/thermal treatment, 1971 tonnes of incineration/insignificant fuel value; 5311 tonnes for wastewater treat-ment and 147 tonnes to waste broker-waste treatment. A total of 493 980 tonnes of methanol was treated, consisting of 260 875 tonnes treated on-site and 197 400 tonnes off-site. A total of 1510 tonnes of methanol was released to land, primarily to on-site landfills (US EPA, 1994).

The total amount of methanol release in Canada in 1993 was 306 222 tonnes distributed as follows: air, 15 326; water, 14 248; underground, 819 and land, 205 (Ministry of Supply & Services Canada, 1993).

Tail pipe emissions as well as evaporative emissions are monitored by a number of agencies. Emissions and air quality modelling results have been reported from methanol/gasoline blends in prototype flexible/variable fuelled vehicles (US EPA, 1991; Auto/Oil Air Quality Research Program, 1992, 1994). Motor vehicle emissions are affected in various ways by the use of methanol fuels in production flexible/variable fuel vehicles. Higher molecular weight hydrocarbons are reduced and carbon monoxide is reduced under some circumstances, while increases in methanol and formaldehyde can occur (US EPA, 1991).

Methanol has been found in significant amounts in the exhaust from gasoline-powered vehicles as well as in diesel exhausts. Methanol was measured at levels of 100-226 mg/kg in the exhaust emissions from non-catalyst vehicles fuelled with isobutane/methanol/gasoline (2/15/83; M-15). Methanol emissions from a light-duty diesel vehicle fuelled with 95% methanol were one order of magnitude higher (3.4 g/kg) (Jonsson et al., 1985).

Chang & Rudy (1990) reported methanol emission factors for vehicles fuelled by M-85 (85% methanol + 15% gasoline) and M-100 (100% methanol) in the USA. For M-85-fuelled vehicles, factors were 0.156-0.7 g methanol/mile driven in exhaust emissions and 0.055-0.25 g methanol/mile driven in evaporative emissions. For M-100 fuelled vehicles, they were 0.5 g methanol/mile driven in exhaust emissions and 0.072-0.134 g methanol/mile driven in evaporative emissions.

Methanol was found at levels of 130-800 $\mu g/m^3$ (0.1 to 0.6 ppm) in the exhaust from nine hydrocarbon test fuels, e.g., iso-octane, iso-octene, benzene, 2-methyl-2-butene, toluene, *o*-xylene, benzene/*n*-pentane, toluene/*n*-pentane and iso-octane/toluene/iso-octene (Seizinger & Dimitriades, 1972).

Methanol, formaldehyde and hydrocarbon emissions from methanol-fuelled cars were reported by Williams et al. (1990). The variable methanol-fuelled vehicles using fuel mixtures of 100, 85, 50, 15 and 0% methanol and a dedicated methanol vehicle all gave similar emission patterns. The organic composition of the exhaust was 85-90% methanol, 5-7% formaldehyde and 3-9% hydrocarbons.

4. ENVIRONMENTAL TRANSPORT, DISTRIBUTION AND TRANSFORMATION

4.1 Transport and distribution between media

Methanol is released into the environment from both natural and man-made sources, the latter being the most significant. Methanol is released predominantly from its production and use as a solvent in industrial processes (in extraction, washing, drying and recrystallization operations), and to a lesser degree from a variety of industrial processes and domestic uses (US EPA, 1980a,b; Graedel et al., 1986; CEC, 1988; Howard, 1990; Nielsen et al., 1993).

Methanol volatilization half-lives of 5.3 and 2.6 days have been estimated for a model river (1 m deep) and an environmental pond, respectively (Howard, 1990).

Methanol is expected to exist almost entirely in the vapour phase in the ambient atmosphere, based on its vapour pressure (Eisenreich et al., 1981; Graedel et al., 1986). Because of methanol's water solubility, rain would be expected to physically remove some methanol from the air (US EPA, 1980a,b; Snider & Dawson, 1985).

Methanol has been found in the atmosphere (Graedel et al., 1986). It can be the product of atmospheric alkane chemistry with concentrations as high as 131 $\mu g/m^3$ (100 ppb) being found. Methanol is expected to become an important additional trace gas in the atmosphere due to its projected increased use as an alternative fuel to gasoline or in a gasoline blend (CEC, 1988; Chang & Rudy, 1990).

The miscibility of methanol in water and its low octanol/water partition coefficient suggest high mobility in soil. Løkke (1984) studied the adsorption of methanol onto three soil types at 6 °C. The soils tested comprised two sandy soils (organic matter contents of 0.09 and 0.1%), and a clay soil (organic matter content of 0.22%). Methanol solutions with concentrations of 0.1, 1.0, 9 and 90 mg/litre were used in 1-h exposure studies. Adsorption coefficients for all soil methanol concentrations and soil types ranged from 0.13 to 0.61, indicating methanol has a low adsorptive capacity on these soils. However Nielsen et al. (1993) suggested that the soils used in the Løkke (1984) study had low organic matter contents compared to typical agricultural surface soil which can have organic matter contents of 1 to 2%, and up to 5% in some soils. A soil containing a typical amount of organic matter might therefore be expected to retain methanol and prevent it from reaching the subsoil.

Additionally, the relatively high vapour pressure and low adsorptive capacity suggests significant evaporation from dry surfaces.

4.2 Transformation

4.2.1 Biodegradation

Methanol is readily biodegradable in soil and sediments, both under aerobic and anaerobic conditions. A large number of strains/ genera of microorganisms have been identified as capable of using methanol as a growth substrate (Hanson, 1980; Braun & Stolp, 1985; Nielsen et al., 1993). These include *Pseudomonas* sp., *Methylobacterium organophilium; Hyphomicrobium* sp., *Desulfovibrio; Streptomyces* sp., *Rhodopseudomonas acidophilia; Paracoccus denitrificans; Microcyclus aquaticus; Thiobacillus novellus; Micrococcus denitrificans; Achromobacter 1L* (isolated from activated sewage sludge) and *Mycobacterium 50* (isolated from activated sewage sludge). Most microorganisms possess the enzyme alcohol dehydrogenase which is necessary for methanol oxidation. The methanogen, *Methanosarcine barkeri* can grow on and produce methane from methanol (Hippe et al., 1979).

The following genera of methanol-oxidizing yeasts have been reported: *Pichia; Saccharomyces; Hansenula; Rhodotorula; Kloechera; Candida; Torulopsis* (Stensel et al., 1973; Hanson, 1980; Nielsen et al., 1993). Okpokwasili & Amanchukwu (1988) isolated *Candida* sp. from Niger Delta sediment which utilized methanol as a growth substrate.

4.2.1.1 Water and sewage sludge

In a closed bottle test, according to OECD guideline 301D, methanol was found to be readily biodegradable with 99% COD removal after the test period of 30 days (Hüls AG, 1978). In another closed bottle test using unadapted inoculum from domestic sewage the degradation of methanol at concentrations of 3, 7 or 10 mg/litre in both freshwater (settled domestic wastewater) and synthetic seawater incubated for a maximum of 20 days under aerobic conditions was studied by Price et al. (1974). Methanol was readily degraded in both inocula at all concentrations with average disappearance of methanol as follows: a) after 5 days, 76% bio-oxidation in fresh water and 69% in salt water; b) after 10 days, 88% bio-oxidation in fresh water and 84% in salt water; c) after 15 days, 91% bio-oxidation in fresh water and 85% in salt water and d) after 20 days, 95% bio-oxidation in fresh water and 97% in salt water.

Matsui et al. (1988) studied the biodegradability of methanol in a batch reactor using activated sludge from an industrial wastewater treatment plant which was acclimatized to the wastewater originating from a petrochemical complex in Japan. Methanol at an initial concentration of 100 mg/litre and an acclimation period of 1 day was found to be highly biodegradable with 91% COD removal and 92% TOC removal achieved.

Incubation of 0.05 mg methanol/litre for 5 days in activated sludge from a municipal sewage plant resulted in the degradation of 37% of the methanol (Freitag et al., 1985). Hatfield (1957) found that at a feed rate of 333 or 500 mg/litre, methanol was virtually completely oxidized (with a major portion of the BOD and COD removed) by acclimated microorganisms within 6 h in a settled domestic sewage inoculum.

The microbial metabolism of methanol in a model activated sludge system monitored by Swain & Somerville (1978) revealed that methanol was not broken down when added transiently (0.23% by volume) to the system operating with a retention time of 11 h. However adaptation of the sludge in such a system to 0.1% by volume occurred over a period of several days. After 2 days acclimation, about 50% of the methanol was utilized, and after 6 days acclimation more than 80% of the methanol had been metabolized. There were no apparent toxic effects caused by the addition of methanol (0.1% by volume) to the sludge prior to and after adaptation to methanol.

The anaerobic treatment of wastes containing methanol and higher alcohols (approximately 50:50 mix) was studied by Lettinga et al. (1981). In batch and continuous experiments using an inoculum consisting of sugar beet waste and active anaerobic sludge, the breakdown of methanol began within a few days while the breakdown of higher alcohols occurred immediately depending on the initial load of waste applied.

Denitrification is facilitated by heterotrophic and autotrophic bacteria. Heterotrophic bacteria require a carbon source for their growth and cell metabolism which can be supplied by methanol (Stensel et al., 1973; Nyberg et al., 1992; Jansen et al., 1993; Upton, 1993). Bacteria such as the organisms of the genera *Pseudomonas, Micrococcus, Achromobacter, Spirillum*, and *Bacillus* reduce nitrate, nitrogen oxide and nitrous oxide under anaerobic conditions. The addition of methanol to promote denitrification has been suggested in situations where nitrate accumulates, and methanol has been added as an economic exogenous organic carbon source to increase denitrification (Stensel et al., 1973; Nyberg et al., 1992; Jansen et al., 1993; Upton, 1993).

At a wastewater treatment plant in Malmo, Sweden, complete denitrification was obtained after approximately one month at 10 °C after methanol was added for denitrification. Microscopic examination revealed a growing population of budding and/or appendaged bacteria, presumably *Hyphomicrobrium spp.* reaching a stable maximum at the time when optimal nitrate removal occurred (Nyberg et al., 1992)

Upton (1993) described a pilot study in the United Kingdom indicating that denitrification in deep-bed sand filters is a feasible technology utilizing methanol addition. Nitrogen removals greater than 70% were possible at winter sewage temperatures.

Several other laboratory studies using a variety of methodologies have demonstrated the rapid biodegradation of methanol by sewage organisms. These show degradation of between 66 and 95%, and usually greater than 80%, within five days (Kempa, 1976; Hüls AG, 1978; Matsui et al., 1988).

4.2.1.2 Soils and sediments

Methanol is biodegradable in soils and sediments, both under aerobic and anaerobic conditions. Methanol is a normal growth substrate for many soil microorganisms, which are capable of completely mineralizing methanol to carbon monoxide and water (CEC, 1988; Howard, 1990; Howard et al., 1991; Nielsen et al., 1993). Methanol at concentrations of up to 1000 mg/litre was degraded to non-measurable amounts within a year or less in subsurface soil and ground water sites in Pennsylvania, New York and Virginia (USA) believed to be previously uncontaminated. Complete degradation of 100 g methanol/litre occurred in less than 30 days in one aerobic soil sample from a Pennsylvania site (Novak et al., 1985).

Scheunert et al. (1987) monitored the formation of $^{14}CO_2$ from labelled methanol in aerobic and anaerobic suspended soil and found methanol to be readily degradable after 5 days incubation at 35 °C. Rates and patterns of biodegradation of methanol in surface and subsurface soils from eight sites in New York, Pennsylvania and Virginia in static microcosms under anaerobic conditions were evaluated by Hickman & Novak (1989) and Hickman et al. (1989). The rates of methanol degradation varied considerably between sites, but the soils could be characterized into two general types, namely fast soils, in which degradation rates were high and rates were increased by addition of nitrate and sulfate, and slow soils, in which biodegradation rates were low and decreased by the addition of nitrate or sulfate and inhibition of sulfate increased degradation rates. Biodegradation rates in subsurface soils were generally within the range of 0.5-1.1 mg/litre per day and indicated that no acclimation period was required. Biodegradation rates were calculated and used to estimate a half-life of between 58 and 263 days for methanol in these soils (Hickman et al., 1989).

Compared to other substrates studied, e.g., acetate, trimethylamine and methylamine, methanol (at concentrations less than 3 µM) was degraded relatively slowly mainly to carbon dioxide, principally via sulfite-reducing organisms, and could not be considered a significant *in situ* precursor in surface sediments of an intertidal zone in Maine, USA (King et al., 1983).

Methanol was found to be an important substrate for methanogenic bacteria in anaerobic sediments (highly reduced and containing methane and hydrogen sulfide), collected from a salt marsh located in San Francisco Bay, California. The sediments were homogenized anaerobically with San Francisco Bay water and 310-340 µmol methanol/flask, resulting in 83-91% conversion to methane, carbon dioxide and water after 3 days (Oremland et al., 1982).

A sulfate-reducing bacterium of the genus *Desulfovibrio*, which is capable of degrading methanol after growth on pyruvate, malate or fumarate, completely converted anaerobic samples of ^{14}C-methanol to carbon dioxide. However the ^{14}C-label was not used as a carbon source by the bacterium and was not assimilated into cellular material (Braun & Stolp, 1985).

4.2.2 Abiotic degradation

4.2.2.1 Water

In a 5-day experiment, ^{14}C-labelled methanol applied to soil-water suspensions under both aerobic and anaerobic conditions yielded 53.4 and 46.3% ^{14}CO$_2$, respectively (Scheunert et al., 1987).

Half-lives of 5.1 years and 46.6 days for the photooxidation of methanol in water have been reported based on the measured rate data for the reaction with hydroxyl radicals in aqueous solutions (Howard et al., 1991). A bimolecular reaction rate constant of 8.5 x 10^{-13} cm^3/molecule per second for the reaction of methanol and hydroxyl radicals in water has been reported by Lemaire et al. (1982).

The rate constant for the reaction of methanol with hydroxyl radicals in aqueous solution is approximately 1 x 10^9 litre/mol per second (Gurten et al., 1984). If the hydroxyl radical concentration of sunlit natural water is assumed to be 1 x 10^{-17} mol/litre (Mill et al., 1980), the half-life of methanol would be approximately 2.2 years (Howard, 1990).

Sediment and clay suspensions did not photo-catalyse the degradation of methanol in aqueous solution during ultraviolet irradiation at 300 nm. However, the addition of semi-conductor powders such as titanium dioxide led to large increases in the yield of formaldehyde upon irradiation, in contrast to the small amounts of formaldehyde formed from the irradiation of 10% aqueous methanol (Oliver et al., 1979).

Hustert et al. (1981) reported that methanol in aqueous solution was stable when exposed to sunlight. Alcohols are generally resistant to environmental aqueous hydrolysis (Lyman et al., 1982; Howard, 1990).

2.2.2   *Air*

Methanol reacts in the atmosphere with oxidizing species (Barnes et al., 1982; Lemaire et al., 1982; Whitbeck, 1983; Graedel et al., 1986; Montgomery, 1991; Nielsen et al., 1993; US EPA, 1994).

The atmospheric lifetime of methanol has been estimated to be 20 days based on the reaction of compounds with the hydroxyl radical, and assuming a hydroxyl free radical concentration of 5×10^5 radicals/cm^3 (Graedel et al., 1986). Methanol half-lives of 8.4 days (US EPA, 1979), 8.0 days (Lemaire et al., 1982) and 7.3 days (Barnes et al., 1982) have also been reported based on reactions at 300 °K and equations reported in Lyman et al. (1984) and Resenblatt (1990). Gusten et al. (1984) reported that at 300 °K and atmospheric pressure, an average hydroxyl concentration of 1×10^6 molecules/cm^3 and a reaction rate constant of 0.95×10^{-12} cm^3/mol per sec, the half-life of methanol was 8.4 days.

Reaction of methanol with nitrogen dioxide in a smog chamber yielded methyl nitrite and nitric acid and the surface reaction of methanol and nitrogen dioxide was enhanced under ultraviolet light (Akimoto & Takagi, 1986). The reaction of methanol with nitrogen dioxide may be the major source of methyl nitrite found in polluted atmospheres (Takagi et al., 1986; Howard, 1990). Only 4.1% of the methanol applied to silica gel was degraded when irradiated for 17 h at wavelengths greater than 290 nm (Freitag et al., 1985).

4.2.3   **Bioconcentration**

Bioconcentration factors (BCFs) of methanol experimentally measured in aquatic organisms using a log k_{ow} value for methanol of -0.77 and correlation equations reported in Lyman et al. (1990) ranged from 0.01-0.51 (Nielsen et al., 1993). Based on the octanol/water partition coefficient of -0.77, the BCF value for methanol was estimated to be 0.2 (Howard, 1990).

Freitag et al. (1985) reported a BCF of < 10 (wet weight basis) for the golden ide (*Leuciscus idus melanotus*) after 3 days exposure to 0.05 mg methanol/litre.

Gluth et al. (1985) proposed a BCF of about 1 for the carp *Cyprinus carpio* exposed to ^{14}C-methanol for up to 72 h. The amount of radioactivity was measured in the liver, kidneys, intestine, muscle, blood and gills of carp exposed to methanol at 5 mg/litre. The initial uptake of methanol into the different tissue types was the same after 24 h and levels remained constant for over 72 h in the liver, kidneys, gills and intestines, but dropped slightly in the blood and muscle.

Geyer et al. (1984) calculated a BCF of 28 400 (dry weight. basis) for the green alga *Chlorella fusca* exposed to 0.05 mg/litre ^{14}C-labelled methanol for 24 h at a temperature of 20-25 °C with 16 h illumination and with agitation. Nielsen et al. (1993) suggested that this high bioconcentration factor is anomalous compared to those for other aquatic organisms. It may be due to the fact that methanol is metabolized by the algae, and the ^{14}C-label, which is measured to calculate the BCF value, is incorporated into the algae in metabolic forms other than methanol.

5. ENVIRONMENTAL LEVELS AND HUMAN EXPOSURE

5.1 Environmental levels

5.1.1 Air

Methanol was detected at mean ambient concentrations of 10 and 3 $\mu g/m^3$ (7.9 and 2.6 ppb) at Tucson, Arizona, USA, and two remote Arizona locations, respectively, during monitoring in 1982 of air pollutants in the USA (Snider & Dawson, 1985). It was also detected in rural air in Alabama (Holzer et al., 1977). Methanol was detected at concentrations of 0.65-1.8 $\mu g/m^3$ (0.5-1.2 ppb) (average 0.77 ppb methanol plus ethanol) in Arctic air from Point Barrow, Alaska, in September 1967 (Cavanaugh et al., 1969).

Urban air levels of methanol in the range of 10.5-131 $\mu g/m^3$ (8-100 ppb) have been reported (Graedel et al., 1986). Jonsson et al. (1985) reported significant amounts of methanol (0.59-94 $\mu g/m^3$; 0.45-72 ppb) at dense traffic sites in Stockholm, Sweden. Average ambient methanol concentrations of 5-30 $\mu g/m^3$ (3.83-26.7 ppb) were detected at five sites in and around Stockholm.

In 1994, methanol was listed as one of the 189 hazardous air pollutants (HAPs) under the Clean Air Act Amendment of 1990, Title III in the USA (Kelly et al., 1994). In a US EPA (1993) summary, median methanol levels of 6-60 $\mu g/m^3$ were found in 52 samples from three locations (Boston, Houston, and Lima, Ohio) in the USA.

5.1.2 Water

Data on the occurrence of methanol in water, particularly finished drinking-water, is limited. Methanol was identified in water at 24 locations in the USA during the period 1974-1976 (US EPA, 1976b). The frequency of occurrence was as follows: finished drinking-water, 12; effluents from chemical plants, 6; effluents from sewage treatment, 4; effluents from paper production, 1; and effluents from latex production, 1.

Methanol was detected in the USA at a mean level of 22 µg/litre in rainwater collected during a thunderstorm in Arizona in 1982 (Snider & Dawson, 1985).

Methanol at levels of 17-80 mg/litre (17-80 ppm) was detected in wastewater effluents from a speciality chemicals manufacturing facility in Massachusetts, USA, but none was detected in associated river water or sediments (Jungclaus et al., 1978). A concentration of 42.4 mg/litre were found in a leachate from the Love Canal in Niagara Falls, New York (Venkataraman et al., 1984). Methanol at a level of 1050 mg/litre was detected in condensate waters discharged from a coal gasification plant at North Dakota, USA (Mohr & King, 1985).

5.1.3   Food

Dietary methanol can arise in large part from fresh fruits and vegetables where it occurs as the free alcohol, methyl esters of fatty acids or methoxy group on polysaccharides such as pectin (Kirchner & Miller, 1957; Casey et al., 1963; Self et al., 1963; Lund et al., 1981; Stegink et al., 1981; Monte, 1984).

The methanol content of fresh and canned fruit juices (principally orange and grapefruit juices) varies considerably and may range from 1-43 mg/litre (Kirchner & Miller, 1957), 10-80 mg/litre (Lund et al., 1981; Monte, 1984) and 12-640 mg/litre with an average of 140 mg/litre (Francot & Geoffroy, 1956; Monte, 1984). Methanol evolved during the cooking of high pectin foods (Casey et al., 1963) has been accounted for in the volatile fraction during boiling and is quickly lost to the atmosphere (Self et al., 1963). However entrapment of the volatiles during canning is possible and probably accounts for the elevated methanol levels of certain fruits and vegetables during this process (Lund et al., 1981).

Fermented distilled beverages can contain high levels of methanol, with some neutral spirits having as much as 1.5 g/litre (Francot & Geoffroy, 1956). Methanol was found at levels of 6-27 mg/litre in beer, 96-321 mg/litre in wines and 10-220 mg/litre in distilled spirits (Greizerstein, 1981). The methanol content in representative beverage alcohol varied between 40 and 55 mg/litre bourbon. This value is comparable with those reported by the distillers. The concentration of methanol in 50% grain alcohol was found to be approximately 1 mg/litre (Majchrowicz & Mendelson, 1971).

The presence of methanol in distilled spirits is directly linked to the pectin content of the raw materials. During the process of making fruit spirits, pectic substances contained in different parts of the fruit undergo degradation by pectin methylases, which can lead to the formation of significant quantities of methanol (Bindler et al., 1988). Concentrations of methanol permitted in brandies in the USA, Canada and Italy range from 6-7 g/litre ethanol (Bindler et al., 1988).

Methanol has been identified in the volatile fraction of sherry wine vinegars (Blanch et al., 1992), lemon, orange and lime extracts, distilled liquors and cordials (AOAC, 1980, 1990).

Methanol has been identified as a volatile component of dried legumes with reported levels of 1.5-7.9 mg/kg in beans, 3.6 mg/kg in split peas and 4.4 mg/kg in lentils (Lovegren et al., 1979). Methanol has also been reported (no levels stated) in roasted filberts (Kinlin et al., 1972) and baked potatoes (Coleman et al., 1981). It has been detected in low-boiling volatile fractions of cooked foods, including Brussels sprouts, carrots, celery, corn, onion, parsnip, peas and potatoes (Self et al., 1963).

Humans can also ingest varying amounts of methanol in foods and or drugs isolated or recrystallized from methanol, e.g., methanol is used as an extraction solvent for spice oleoresins and hops (Lewis, 1989). Additionally, certain foods and drugs, consumed or administered as their methyl ester, can release methanol during their metabolism and excretion (Stegink et al., 1981; Davoli et al., 1986). For example, 10% of the sweetening agent aspartame (L-aspartyl-L-phenylalanine methyl ester) hydrolyzes in the gastrointestinal tract to become free methanol. Carbonated beverages contain about 555 mg aspartame/litre (Medinsky & Dorman, 1994), equivalent to approximately 56 mg methanol per litre.

The amount of methanol present in an average serving of beverage sweetened by aspartame alone is considerably less than in the same volume of many fruit and vegetable juices. For instance, tomato juice will result in 6 times the amount of methanol exposure than consumption of an equivalent volume of aspartame sweetened beverage (Wucherpfennig et al., 1983).

Exposure to several industrial compounds such as methanol, formaldehyde and acetone may contribute to increasing amounts of formate in the body (Boeniger, 1987). Formate is present in blood at background or endogenous levels that range from 0.07 to 0.4 mM. Although it is essential for survival, an excess of formate, which often occurs after intake of large doses of methanol, can cause severe toxicity and even death (Medinsky & Dorman, 1994).

Ingestion of formate can arise from such foods as honey, fruit syrups and roasted coffee as well as from its use as a food preservative. Formate is also produced as a by-product of several metabolic pathways including histidine and tryptophan degradation (Stegink et al., 1983).

The possible utility of formic acid as a biomarker for occupational exposure to methanol has been investigated (Angerer & Lehnert, 1977; Baumann & Angerer, 1979; Ferry et al., 1980; Heinrich & Angerer, 1982; Liesivouri & Savolainen, 1987; Franzblau et al., 1992b; Lee et al., 1992; d'Alessandro et al., 1994).

5.1.4   *Tobacco smoke*

Methanol at levels of 180 µg/cigarette has been detected in the vapour phase in mainstream smoke (Norman, 1977; Guerin et al., 1987). It has been reported to represent about 2% by weight of the mainstream smoke organic phase and particulate matter (Dube & Green, 1982).

5.2   Occupational exposure

US NIOSH (1976) estimated that 175 000 workers in the USA are potentially exposed to methanol. As stated in Clayton & Clayton (1982), the US Department of Labor reported that 72 occupations involve exposure to methanol. Estimates derived from the NIOSH 1972/1974 National Occupational Hazard Survey and 1982-1983 National Occupational Exposure Survey indicate that approximately 1-2 million workers in the USA are potentially exposed to methanol (Howard, 1990).

In a 1978-1982 survey of solvent products associated with USA industrial workplace exposure, methanol was identified in 9.8% of 275 solvent samples collected. The products represented solvent classes such as thinners, degreasers, paints, inks and adhesives (Howard, 1990).

Workplace concentrations in the range of 29-108 mg/m^3 were found during production of "fused collars" (Greenberg et al., 1938). No signs or symptoms of methanol intoxication were observed.

In the vicinity of "spirit" duplicator machines operated with methanol-based duplicator fluids, methanol concentrations of between 475 to 4000 mg/m^3 were found in the breathing zone. Teacher aides and clerical workers exposed to these concentrations experienced typical symptoms of methanol intoxication (Kingsley & Hirsch, 1955; NIOSH, 1981; Frederick et al., 1984).

In a Japanese factory producing canned fuel containing mainly methanol, air levels of methanol were high (Kawai et al., 1991b). A mean geometric concentration of 600 mg/m^3 (459 ppm) with a geometric standard derivation of 4.1 was found in the breathing zone of 22 production workers (8-h sampling). This resulted in high blood and urine levels of methanol (see section 8.1.3 for further details).

In a chemical plant, 30-min workplace concentrations ranged from about 49 to 303 mg/m^3 during the course of a shift, with a geometric mean of 129 mg/m^3. After an 8-h exposure, average methanol blood and urine levels of 8.9 ± 14.7 and 21.8 ± 20.0 mg/litre and a mean formic acid urine level of 29.9 ± 28.6 mg/litre were found (Heinrich & Angerer, 1982).

Increases in blood and urine methanol and formate levels can be measured in humans exposed to methanol vapours in the workplace at concentrations below the ACGIH threshold limit value (TLV) of 260 mg/m^3 (200 ppm). The recommended limit of 260 mg/m^3 for methanol was first proposed by Cook (1945), based on previous studies of Sayers et al. (1942) who observed no symptoms in dogs exposed daily (7 days/week) for 379 days at concentrations between 590 and 655 mg/m^3 (450 and 500 ppm). Printing office and chemical workers exposed to approximately 130 mg/m^3 (100 ppm) during the workshift exhibited a 1.5- to 2.5-fold increase in blood and urinary formate and a 15- to 20-fold increase in blood and urinary methanol at the end of the workday, whereas unexposed workers did not exhibit an increase in their blood and urinary methanol or formate levels (Baumann & Angerer, 1979; Heinrich & Angerer, 1982).

5.3 General population

Humans are routinely exposed to methanol from both the diet and natural metabolic processes. Sedivec et al. (1981) reported a mean blood methanol level of 0.73 mg/litre in 31 unexposed subjects (range: 0.32-2.61 mg/litre). Eriksen & Kulkarni (1963) measured a mean level of 0.25 µg/litre in the expired air of 9 "normal" people (range: 0.06-0.45 µg/litre).

Methanol is available from the ingestion of dietary fruits and vegetables, from the consumption of fruit juices and fermentation beverages, and from the use of the synthetic sweetener aspartame, which on hydrolysis yields 10% of its weight as free methanol, which is available for absorption. Estimates of intakes of methanol from these sources vary considerably. Consuming a 354 ml carbonated beverage is approximately equivalent to a methanol intake of 20 mg. Excluding exposure from carbonated beverages, daily aspartame intake can average 3-11 mg/kg (0.3-1.1 mg methanol/kg), with the 99th percentile ingesting up to 34 mg/kg (3.4 mg/kg methanol) (Stegink, 1981; Medinsky & Dorman, 1994). If aspartame were used to replace all sucrose in the diet, its average daily ingestion would be 7.5-8.5 mg/kg which would be the equivalent to 0.75-0.85 mg methanol/kg (Stegink et al., 1981; Davoli et al., 1986).

The average intake of methanol from natural sources varies, but limited data suggest an average intake of considerably less than 10 mg methanol/day (US EPA, 1977; Monte, 1984).

Estimated methanol body burdens for selected situations were reported by Medinsky & Dormam (1994). The "background" body burden of methanol was estimated to be 0.5 mg/kg. Fruit juices containing 12-640 mg methanol/litre would have a variable effect on body burden, while personal garage exposure (200 mg/m^3; 15 min) and self-service refuelling (50 mg/m^3; 4 min) would increase the body burdens by an estimated 0.6 mg/kg and 0.04 mg/kg, respectively.

Methanol, either 100% or in gasoline blends (85% methanol and 15% gasoline), has the potential to become a major automotive fuel particularly in the USA in the next century (Kavet & Nauss, 1990; Medinsky & Dorman, 1994). Emissions of methanol can arise from its release as uncombusted fuel in the exhaust or from its evaporation during refuelling and after the engine has stopped. Formaldehyde emissions can result from the incomplete combustion of methanol fuels (Medinsky & Dorman, 1994).

The US EPA has modelled methanol exposure levels that might occur under specific conditions of use (Kavet & Nauss, 1990). For example, if 100% of all automobiles were powered by methanol-based fuels, models predict concentrations of methanol in expressways, street canyons, railroad tunnels or parking garages ranging from a low of 1 mg/m^3 to a high of 60 mg/m^3. Methanol concentrations in a personal garage during engine idle or hot soak conditions are predicted to range from 2.9 to 50 mg/m^3, while those predicted during refuelling of vehicles ranged from 30 to 50 mg/m^3. For comparison, the American Conference of Governmental Industrial Hygienists (ACGIH) Threshold Limit Value (TLV) for exposure to methanol over an 8-h workday is 260 mg/m^3 (200 ppm) for working populations.

Some methanol exposure concentrations have been calculated for various scenarios (traffic conditions, wind patterns, meteorological conditions) from emission data from a few cars using methanol dispersion models. The highest methanol concentration projected to occur in a personal garage is 490 mg/m^3 (375 ppm) during the cold start. In public garages, assuming 100% of the vehicles were fuelled with methanol, concentrations were projected to be as high as 200 mg/m^3 (150 ppm), while in either scenarios the concentrations would be expected to be lower than 65 mg/m^3 (50 ppm). In the majority of cases, exposure to the general public would be brief but repeated in time (Gold & Moulif, 1988).

Most available evidence indicates that exposure to methanol vapour from use as a motor fuel is not associated with adverse effects (Gold & Moulif, 1988). The uncertainties in this conclusion are based on the lack of information at reasonable projected exposure levels and of studies examining end-points of concern in sensitive species. Lack of complete data (dose-response, exposure) reveals that numerous uncertainties exist in the safety/risk assessments. Small effects and trends in behavioural and neurophysiological responses and subjective ratings have been reported but need to be further substantiated.

6. KINETICS AND METABOLISM IN LABORATORY ANIMALS AND HUMANS

6.1 Absorption

The primary routes of methanol exposure are inhalation and ingestion, with dermal exposure currently of much less importance in terms of total daily intake for both the general and occupational populations. Regardless of the exposure route, methanol distributes readily and uniformly to all organs and tissues in direct relation to their water content (Yant & Schrenk, 1937; Haggard & Greenberg, 1939). Thus all exposure routes are presumed to be toxicologically equivalent (Tephly & McMartin, 1984). No differences exist between the capabilities for absorption of methanol among various animal species, and blood levels are entirely predictable based on the concept that methanol distributes uniformly to body water content.

6.1.1 Inhalation

Inhalation of methanol is the most common route of entry in an occupational setting. Experiences in occupational health and volunteer studies show that methanol is rapidly absorbed after inhalation (Angerer & Lehnert, 1977; Baumann & Angerer, 1979; Ferry et al., 1980; Sedivec et al., 1981; Heinrich & Angerer, 1982; Liesivouri & Savolainen, 1987; Kawai et al., 1992; d'Alessandro et al., 1994).

The body burden is estimated from methanol concentration, ventilation rate, duration of exposure and lung retention. Around 60-85% of inhaled methanol is absorbed in the lung of humans (Leaf & Zatman, 1952; Sedivec et al., 1981). Blood methanol concentration, frequently employed to characterize the body burden of methanol is, on average, equal to 83% of its aqueous concentration. Urine contains methanol concentrations 20-30% higher than blood (Yant & Schrenk, 1937; Leaf & Zatman, 1952).

Following uptake and distribution, methanol clears from the body. In humans, clearance proceeds after either inhalation or oral exposure with a half-life of 1 day or more for high doses (greater than 1 g/kg) and about 3 h for low doses (less than 0.1 g/kg) with first-order kinetics in humans, monkeys and rats (Leaf & Zatman, 1952; Teply & McMartin, 1984).

Methanol is either excreted unchanged in the urine and breath or it enters a metabolic pathway whose ultimate product is carbon dioxide. The time course for the disappearance of methanol from the circulation is dependent upon the combined action of both direct excretion and metabolism. The elimination of methanol from the blood appears to be very slow in all species, especially when compared to ethanol (Tephly & McMartin, 1984).

Relationships between methanol inhalation exposure, concentrations, duration of exposure and urinary methanol concentrations have been characterized in exposures of volunteers and in occupational settings. Ferry et al. (1980), Sedivec et al. (1981), and Heinrich & Angerer (1982) reported that urinary methanol concentrations strictly depend on the duration and intensity of the methanol exposure, suggesting that measurement of urinary methanol concentrations would be a reliable parameter for evaluating the degree of methanol exposure.

Sedivec et al. (1981) exposed four volunteers to methanol at concentrations of 102, 205 and 300 mg/m^3 for 8 h/day. Urine was monitored for methanol during exposure and for 18 h afterwards. The concentrations in urine were proportional to the air concentrations. When exposure ceased, urinary methanol levels decreased exponentially with a half-life of about 1.5-2 h; a mean urinary level of 0.73 mg/litre (range 0.32-2.61 mg/litre) in 31 unexposed subjects was also reported. Heinrich & Angerer (1982) determined methanol in blood and urine and formic acid in urine from 20 subjects occupationally exposed to methanol. The air concentration was on average 145 mg/m^3 (111 ppm) but varied from 49 to 303 mg/m^3. An 8-h exposure resulted in methanol levels in blood and urine of 8.9 ± 14.7 mg/litre and 21.8 ± 20 mg/litre, respectively. Formic acid concentrations were 29.9 ± 28.6 mg/litre. The corresponding normal values were < 0.6, 1.1 ± 0.9 and 12.7 ± 11.7 mg/litre.

Volunteers exposed for 6 h to 260 mg/m^3 (200 ppm) methanol, the current permissible US OSHA 8-h time-weighted average limit, were found to have a blood methanol concentration increase from a mean of 1.8 µg/ml to 7.0 µg/ml (3.5-4 fold increase) compared to their pre-exposure levels. Formate did not accumulate in the blood above its background level (8.11 µg/ml) following the 6-h exposure (Lee et al., 1992).

Franzblau et al. (1993) demonstrated the absence of formic acid accumulation in the urine of five volunteers following 5 days of exposure to an atmosphere containing 260 mg/m^3 (200 ppm) of methanol in a test chamber. These results indicated that there was no day-to-day accumulation of formic acid in urine in conjunction with 5 consecutive days of near-maximal permissible airborne methanol exposure and that measurement of formic acid in urine specimens collected 16 h following cessation of exposure did not appear to reflect inhalation methanol exposure on the preceding day.

Twenty-six volunteers exposed at rest to 260 mg/m^3 (200 ppm) of methanol vapour for 4 h did not show significant differences in serum or urinary formate concentration. At the TLV of 260 mg/m^3 (200 ppm) methanol exposure did not contribute substantially to endogenous formate formation (d'Alessandro et al., 1994).

Inhalation of from 650 to 1450 mg/m^3 (500 to 1100 ppm) methanol for periods of 3-4 h in humans yielded urine concentrations of about 10-30 mg/litre at the end of the exposure period (Leaf & Zatman, 1952). Based on their findings, it was suggested that an 8-h exposure to 3990 mg/m^3 (3000 ppm) methanol would be necessary before a gradual accumulation of methanol would occur in the body.

6.1.2   Oral

Methanol is rapidly absorbed from the gastrointestinal tract with peak absorption occurring in 30-60 min depending on the presence or absence of food in the stomach (Becker, 1983).

Ingestion of methanol has been the principal route of exposure in the many reported cases of acute poisoning (Buller & Wood, 1904; Wood & Buller, 1904; Bennett et al., 1953; Erlanson et al., 1965; Kane et al., 1968; Gonda et al., 1978; Naraqi et al., 1979; Swartz et al., 1981; Jacobsen et al., 1982; Becker, 1983; Litovitz et al., 1988).

During methanol poisoning in humans, concentrations of methanol and formic acid in blood and urine are quite variable. Concentrations of both compounds are highly dependent upon dose, time following exposure and concomitant ingestion of ethanol (Lund, 1948a, Gonda et al., 1978, Jacobsen et al., 1982a). Excretion of methanol in urine is initially high and decreases with time following exposure. Maximum excretion of formic acid in urine may occur as late as the second or third day following ingestion (Lund, 1948a).

Blood methanol concentrations during experimentally induced ethanol intoxication in alcoholics during a 10-15 day period of chronic alcohol intake showed that blood methanol levels increased progressively from 2-27 mg/litre from the first to the 11th day of drinking, when blood ethanol concentrations ranged between 1500 and 4500 mg/litre. Blood methanol levels decreased at the rate of 2.9 ± 0.4 mg/litre per h only after blood ethanol levels decreased to 700 to 200 mg/litre. Blood methanol disappearance lagged behind the linear disappearance of ethanol by approximately 6-8 h and complete clearance of methanol required several days. Methanol probably accumulates in the blood as a result of the competitive inhibition of alcohol dehydrogenase by ethanol and the presence of endogenously formed methanol (Majchrowicz & Mendelson, 1971).

Oral doses of 71-84 mg methanol/kg in humans resulted in blood levels of 47-76 mg/litre blood 2-3 h later. The urinary concentrations of methanol rapidly reached a peak capacity in 1 h and declined exponentially, reaching control values in 13-16 h. The urine/blood concentration ratio was found to be relatively constant at 0.30 (Leaf & Zatman, 1952). Leaf & Zatman (1952) monitored methanol disappearance from the circulation of three volunteers orally administered 3, 5 and 7 ml (2.4, 4.0 and 5.6 g) (highest dose, 0.08 g/kg). Blood and urine methanol disappearance obeyed first-order kinetics with a half-time of about 3 h.

Aspartame (see section 5.1.3) is a widely used artificial sweetening agent which is hydrolysed in the intestinal mucosa to 10% methanol by weight. Beverages totally sweetened with aspartame typically contain 0.5-0.6 mg aspartame/ml or approximately 195 mg/350 ml soft-drink; dry mixes and puddings use about 100 mg/serving and pre-sweetened cereal products about 60 mg/25 ml (cup). The methanol body burden following ingestion of any of these products could vary from 6-20 mg (Stegink et al., 1981,1983). Clearance of methanol from human circulation after body burdens as high as 80 mg/kg follows first-order kinetics with a half-time of about 2.5-3 h (the rate constant for total clearance k_t is 0.23-0.28/h (Stegink et al., 1981; Kavet & Nauss, 1990).

After intake of small quantities of methanol (10-20 ml), human subjects showed no methanol in blood after 48 h, and the concentration of formic acid in the urine was normal (6.5-12.8 mg%) within 24 h (Lund, 1948a). Following intake of large amounts of methanol (50 ml), methanol was found in the blood (250-1200 mg/litre) after 48 h. Formic acid was found in the blood (26-78 mg/litre) as well as an increased excretion of formic acid in the urine (540-2050 mg/litre), and up to 20 500 mg/litre within 24 h. Maximum excretion of formic acid was found to occur not later than the second or third day after intake of methanol (Lund, 1948a).

6.1.3   *Dermal*

It has been known for some time that pure methanol has an anomalously high diffusion rate through epidermis because of the damage it produces on the stratum corneum (the thin sheath of keratinized cells that comprise the outermost layer of the epidermis). The permeability of epidermis for pure methanol is 10.4 mg/cm^2 per h (Scheuplein & Blank, 1971).

Skin absorption rate studies of methanol ranging from 0.031-0.241 mg/cm^2 per min conducted in human volunteers showed that an average of 0.192 mg methanol/cm^2 per min is absorbed through direct contact of the skin to methanol. Compared with absorption via the respiratory tract, exposure of one hand to liquid methanol for only 2 min would result in a body burden of as much as 170 mg methanol, similar to that resulting from exposure to an approximate air concentration of 50 mg/m^3 (40 ppm) methanol for 8 h (Dutkiewicz et al., 1980). It was also reported that in the context of a 20-min immersion of one hand in methanol, the cumulative urinary excretion of methanol over 8 h was 2 mg. However, it should be noted that the assessment of Dutkiewicz et al. (1980) would imply that a 10-min exposure of one hand to liquid methanol roughly corresponds to an 8-h inhalation exposure at 260 mg/m^3 (200 ppm). Such an inhalation exposure was found to be accompanied with a post-shift urinary methanol concentration of about 40 mg/litre (Sedivec et al., 1981; Kawai et al., 1991b) or 6.5 mg/litre (Franzblau et al., 1993).

The rate of absorption into the skin has been found to be higher with M-85 (85% methanol-15% gasoline) than with pure methanol. The gasoline was suggested to act by drying out the skin allowing the methanol to be more readily absorbed (Machiele, 1990).

In 11 children treated for percutaneous methanol intoxication, methanol blood levels ranged from 0.57 to 11.3 g/litre (mean 4.61 g/litre) (Giminez et al., 1968). Methanol was identified in the urine and in peritoneal fluid (no quantitative estimation) in an 8-month-old boy poisoned by percutaneous absorption of methanol (Kahn & Blum, 1979).

Downie et al. (1992) reported a case of percutaneous industrial methanol toxicity involving two workers who spent 2-3 h cleaning out a cargo tank with methanol while wearing positive pressure breathing apparatus. One of the workers, who suffered from a previous sunburn, wore no protective clothing during cleaning. He experienced methanol toxicity from percutaneous exposure and required hospitalization and methanol poisoning treatment.

6.2 Distribution

Methanol distributes readily and uniformly to organs and tissues in direct relation to their water content (Yant & Schrenk, 1937; Haggard & Greenberg, 1939). The apparent volume of distribution of methanol is 0.6-0.7 litres/kg, similar to that of ethanol. In methanol inhalation studies conducted in dogs, Yang & Schrenk (1937) reported that the highest concentrations of methanol were found in the blood, vitreous and aqueous humour, bile and urine, and the lowest in bone marrow and fatty tissue. In other animal studies, high concentrations of methanol have been reported in the kidney, liver and gastro-intestinal tract with smaller concentrations in brain, muscle and adipose tissue (Bartlett, 1950).

Postmortem analysis of methanol concentrations in body fluids and tissues reported in fatal human cases of methanol poisoning has revealed high concentrations of methanol in cerebrospinal fluid (CSF), vitreous humour and bile (Bennet et al., 1953; Wu Chen, 1985). Methanol concentrations in these fluids were higher than blood concentrations. In one study the ratio of methanol in blood to vitreous humour was 0.82, which was similar to the ratio of ethanol in blood to vitreous humour of 0.89 (Coe & Sherman, 1970). In tissues the highest concentrations were found in brain, kidney, lung and spleen, with lower concentrations in skeletal muscle, pancreas, liver and heart (Wu Chen et al., 1985).

Methanol-induced alterations in uteroplacental blood-flow were studied in CD-1 mice and Sprague-Dawley rats employing microdialysis as a tool for investigating the flux of toxicants across the maternal-conceptual unit. Microdialysis probes were inserted into the uteri of gestational day 20 rats and methanol was administered as either an intravenous bolus (100 or 500 mg/kg) or infusion (100 or 1000 mg/kg/hour).

In separate studies, methanol (100 or 500 mg/kg) and ^3H_2O (20 µCi/kg) were administered intravenously on gestational days 20 and 14 to rats and on gestational day 18 to mice. The methanol concentration-time data were consistent with saturable maternal elimination and apparent first-order transfer between maternal and conceptual compartments. At distribution equilibrium, conceptual methanol concentrations exceeded those in the dam by approximately 25%. The initial rate of conceptual permeation of methanol was proportional to the reciprocal of maternal blood methanol concentration ($r^2 = 0.910$).

The data indicated that high circulating maternal methanol concentrations decrease the rate of presentation of methanol and ^3H_2O to the conceptus, and, depending on the severity of the decrease, fetal hypoxia could also result (Ward & Pollack, 1996b).

6.3 Metabolic transformation

After uptake and distribution, most of the methanol is metabolized in the liver to carbon dioxide (96.9%), while a small fraction is excreted directly to the urine (0.6%) and through the lung. In all mammalian species studied, methanol is metabolized in the liver by sequential oxidative steps to form formaldehyde, formic acid and CO_2 (Fig. 1). However, there are profound differences in the rate of formate oxidation in different species which determine the sensitivity to methanol (Rietbrock, 1969; Palese & Tephly, 1975; McMartin et al., 1977; Eells et al., 1981a, 1983).

Two enzymes are important in the oxidation of methanol to formaldehyde, alcohol dehydrogenase and catalase. In non-human primates and humans, alcohol dehydrogenase mediates this reaction (Makar et al., 1968; Röe, 1982). In rats and other non-primate species this reaction is mediated by catalase. Definitive evidence of these

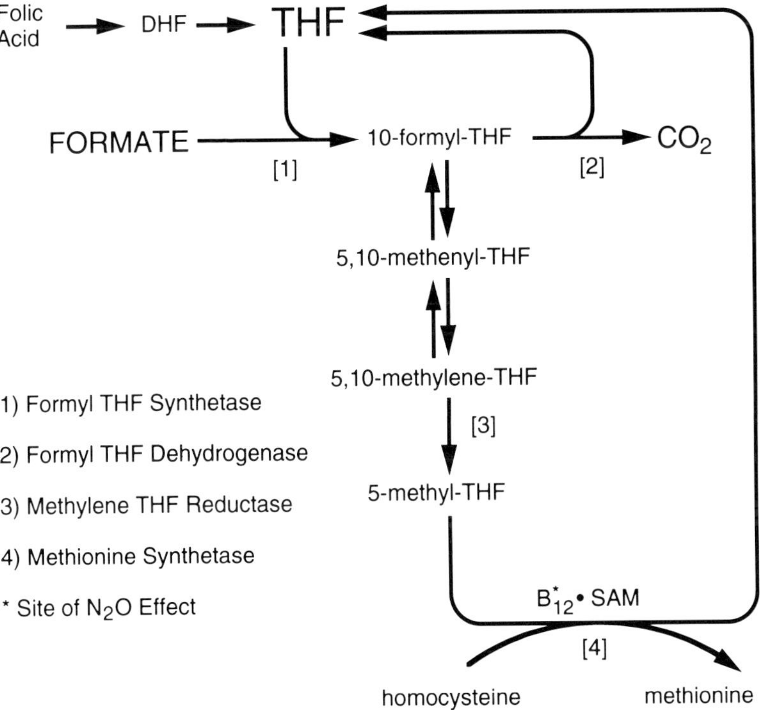

Fig. 1. Metabolism of formate by folate-dependent factors
(from: Eells et al., 1981a)

differences has been provided by studies of methanol oxidation *in vivo* using alternative substrates (ethanol, 1-butanol) and selective inhibitors of catalase (3-amino-1,2,4-triazole) and alcohol dehydrogenase (4-amino-pyrazole). The hepatic microsomal mixed-function oxidase system ($P_{450}IIE1$) has also been implicated in the conversion of methanol to formaldehyde, but there is no definitive information on its role *in vivo* (Rietbrock et al., 1966; Teschke et al., 1975). Despite the difference in enzyme mediation, the conversion from methanol to formate occurs at similar rates in non-human primates and in rats (Tephly et al., 1964; Makar et al., 1968; Noker et al., 1980; Eells et al., 1981a, 1983). The metabolism of methanol can be significantly inhibited by co-exposure to ethanol, which acts as a competing substrate for alcohol dehydrogenase (Jones, 1987).

Formaldehyde is oxidized to formate by several enzyme systems including a specific formaldehyde dehydrogenase. In the reaction catalysed by this enzyme, formaldehyde combines with reduced glutathione to form *S*-formyl glutathione, which is hydrolysed in the presence of thiolase to formate and reduced glutathione (Strittmatter & Ball, 1955; Uotila & Koivusalo, 1974). The second step of this reaction is irreversible (Strittmatter & Ball, 1955). Formaldehyde dehydrogenase activity has been shown to be present in numerous species and tissues including human liver and brain (Strittmatter & Ball, 1955; Kinoshita & Masurat, 1958; Goodman & Tephly, 1971).

The elimination of formaldehyde in many species including primates is extremely rapid with a half-life of approximately 1 min (Rietbrock, 1965; McMartin et al., 1979). Malorny et al. (1965) found that equimolar infusions of formaldehyde, formic acid and sodium formate in dogs produced equivalent peak concentrations of formic acid, indicating that formaldehyde was rapidly metabolized to formic acid. In a human case of formaldehyde poisoning, toxic concentrations of formate (7-8 mm) were detected within 30 min of ingestion, confirming rapid metabolism of formaldehyde to formate in humans (Eells et al., 1981b). Formaldehyde has not been detected in body fluids or tissues following toxic methanol exposures (Makar & Tephly, 1977, McMartin et al., 1977, McMartin et al., 1980a). Formate is oxidized to CO_2 *in vivo* in mammalian species primarily by a tetrahydrofolate-dependent pathway (Fig. 2). Formate enters this pathway by combining with tetrahydrofolate (H_4folate) to form 10-formyl-H_4folate in a reaction catalysed by formyl-tetrahydrofolate synthetase. 10-Formyl-H_4folate may then be further oxidized to CO_2 and H_4folate by formyl-H_4folate dehydrogenase (Kutzbach & Stokstad, 1968) (Fig. 1). Rietbrock et al. (1966) found an inverse correlation between plasma concentrations of folate in different animal species and the half-life of exogenously administered formate, suggesting that folates are involved in formate metabolism. Formate metabolism in rats and monkeys has been shown to be mediated by the folate-

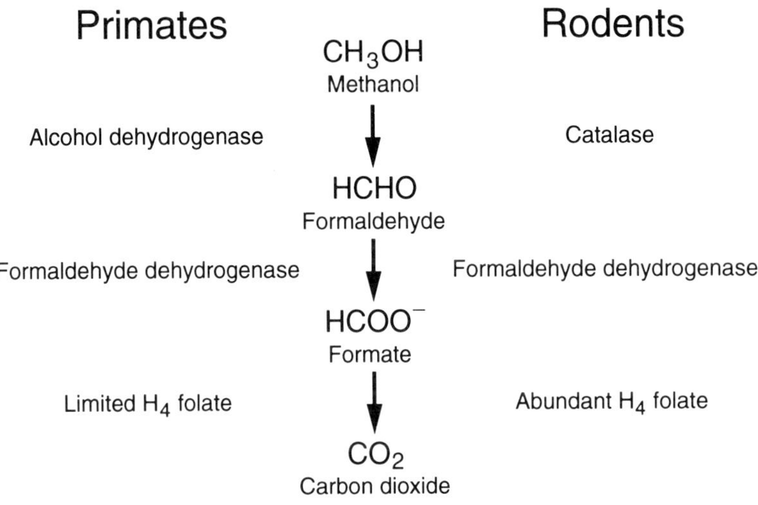

Fig. 2. Scheme for the metabolism of methanol. Major enzymes for primates (left) and rodents (right) are noted. Species differences in methanol toxicity are due primarily to the metabolic conversion of formate to carbon dioxide, which is rapid in rodents but slow in primates (from: Medinsky & Dorman, 1994).

dependent pathway (Makar et al., 1968; Palese & Tephly, 1975). Inhibition of catalase with aminotriazole had no effect on formate oxidation, whereas folate-deficiency markedly reduced formate oxidation in both species. Tetrahydrofolate is derived from folic acid in the diet and is the major determinant of the rate of formate metabolism (McMartin et al., 1975).

The folate-mediated oxidation of formate proceeds about twice as slowly in non-human primates and humans as in rats. This explains the susceptibility of primates to the accumulation of formate, which is seen to occur at doses of methanol greater than 0.5 g/kg (Tephly & McMartin, 1984) (Fig. 2).

There is substantial clinical and experimental evidence that formic acid is the toxic metabolite responsible for the metabolic and visual toxicity characteristic of methanol poisoning. Specifically, formic acid is the toxic metabolite responsible for the metabolic acidosis observed in methanol poisoning in humans, in non-human primates and in folate-depleted rodents (McMartin et al., 1975, 1977, 1980; Eells et al., 1983; Jacobsen & McMartin, 1986; Eells, 1991; Murray et al., 1991; Lee et al., 1994). Formic acid is believed to be the toxic metabolite responsible for the ocular toxicity in methanol-poisoned humans (Sharpe et al., 1982), and is also responsible for the ocular toxicity produced in non-human primates and folate-depleted rodents (Martin-Amat et al., 1977, 1978; Eells et al., 1983; Eells, 1991; Lee et al., 1994a,b).

A comparative metabolism study between rodents and non-human primates showed that formic acid concentration in blood of rats and monkeys was similar at doses of 25, 125 and 600 mg methanol/kg, but became substantially higher in monkeys at 3000 mg/kg. Monkeys and rodents showed different excretion patterns for methanol. As the dose increased, monkeys tended to excrete an increasing percentage of methanol in urine, whereas in rats, the percentage of methanol excreted in expired air increased. Additionally, rats excreted much higher levels of carbon dioxide in expired air (as a percentage of dose) than monkeys (Katoh, 1989).

In a study of formate metabolism in young swine (Makar et al., 1990), it was found that the pig, compared to other species (mouse, rat, monkey and humans), has extremely low levels of hepatic folates. Furthermore, the rate of formate elimination in the pig was much lower in the pig than in the rat. It was suggested that the pig might be sensitive to the methanol toxicity syndrome (metabolic acidosis and blindness).

Ward & Pallack (1996a) studied the *in vitro* biotransformation of methanol in Sprague-Dawley rat and CD-1 mouse fetal livers to assess the capability of the near-term rodent fetus to metabolize methanol. Adult near-term rodent livers metabolized methanol to formate (at gestational day 20) with a maximum of about 85% that in livers from non-pregnant rodents (p < 0.05). This was consistent with *in vivo* experiments (Ward & Pollack, 1996a).

Fetal rat and mouse liver was capable of metabolizing methanol *in vitro*, but only at a rate of < 5% of the respective adult liver. The difference was in fact even greater, considering the difference in organ weight between the conceptus and the dam (about 10-fold).

Fetal mouse liver homogenates converted methanol to formaldehyde at a significantly higher (about 40%) rate than fetal rat liver homogenates. These data suggest that the near-term rodent fetus does not possess a significant ability to biotransform methanol to formaldehyde and ultimately formate *in situ*.

6.4   Elimination and excretion

The primary route of methanol elimination from the body is via oxidation to formaldehyde and then to formic acid, which may be excreted in the urine or further oxidized to carbon dioxide.

In humans, methanol is primarily eliminated by oxidation and only 2% of a 50 mg/kg dose of methanol is excreted unchanged by the lungs and kidney (Leaf & Zatman, 1952). The small excretion of unchanged methanol was also observed in methanol-poisoned subjects in whom the renal and pulmonary excretory clearances of methanol were 1 and 6 ml/min, respectively (Jacobsen et al., 1982a, 1983b).

The elimination of formaldehyde in many species, including primates, is extremely rapid with a half-life of approximately 1 min (McMartin et al., 1979). Toxic concentrations of formate (7-8 mM) were detected within 30 min of ingestion in a human case of formaldehyde poisoning, confirming the rapid metabolism of formaldehyde to formate in humans (Eells et al., 1981b).

Following uptake and distribution methanol is either excreted unchanged (direct excretion) in urine or exhaled breath, or it enters a metabolic pathway in the liver, whose ultimate product is carbon dioxide. The time course of the disappearance of methanol from the circulation is dependent upon the combined action of both direct excretion and metabolism. The clearance from the circulation of humans following low-level exposures to methanol administered orally (<0.1 g/kg) (Leaf & Zatman, 1952) or by inhalation (102-300 mg/m^3) (Sedivec et al., 1981) indicated that methanol disappearance obeyed first-order kinetics with a half-time of about 2.5-3 h in both studies as determined by blood and urinary methanol concentrations. In general estimated methanol dose correlated with resulting blood and urine methanol levels after both ingestion and inhalation, and methanol concentrations in urine were approximately 30% higher than in blood (Leaf & Zatman, 1952).

Elimination half-lives of methanol ranging from 110-213 min were found in human volunteers following consumption of 1000-1500 ml red wine (95% w/w ethanol, 100 mg/litre methanol) the previous evening (Jones, 1987). After concomitant ingestion of a very low dose of methanol (< 2 mg/kg) and ethanol (ethanol: methanol = 10), by human subjects, a 10 fold increase in blood methanol was observed due to the combined ingestion of the alcohols (Jones, 1987). Jacobsen et al. (1982a) reported that during haemolysis in 2 patients being treated for methanol poisoning, the elimination half-lives were 219 and 197 min respectively.

At higher doses of methanol, the elimination appears to become saturated, resulting in nonlinear elimination kinetics. In an untreated methanol-poisoned subject, methanol elimination was clearly zero order with a rate of 85 mg/litre per h, about half the elimination rate of ethanol (Jacobsen et al., 1988). The rates of elimination in two other cases appeared to be 30-50 mg/litre per h (Kane et al., 1968).

The kidney apparently exerts no active control over the urinary concentration of methanol. The methanol content that enters the bladder reflects the aqueous concentration of methanol in the blood (Yant & Schrenk, 1937; Leaf & Zatman, 1952; Sedivec et al., 1981). The rate at which methanol clears into the urine is directly proportional to its blood level which satisfies the condition for first-order kinetics (Kavet & Nauss, 1990).

In the lung, a small fraction of blood-borne methanol is exhaled. The amount of methanol that crosses the blood-air barrier is proportional to its blood concentration (first-order kinetics) and is governed by its blood-air partition ratio (Kavet & Nauss, 1990). In contrast to direct renal and pulmonary excretion, the metabolic conversion of methanol to carbon dioxide is not a linear function of concentration (Tephly et al., 1964; Makar et al., 1968).

Elimination of methanol from the blood appears to be slow in all species especially when compared to ethanol (Tephly & McMartin, 1984; Tephly, 1991).

One to 7 g of methanol/litre of blood (1000-7000 mg/litre) was found in the blood of rats following oral administration of 4 g methanol/kg body weight, and 70% of the methanol lost was eliminated in expired air (Haggard & Greenberg, 1939).

Following administration of a 10% methanol solution (1 g/kg) of ^{14}C-methanol by gavage to the rat, 89% of the administered radioactivity was recovered after 48 h; 65% as CO_2 in expired air, 3% as methanol in urine; 3% as formic acid in urine and 4% fixed in tissues. An oxidation rate of 25 mg/kg/h was found during the first 28 h following methanol administration (Bartlett, 1950a).

Methanol was oxidized at a constant rate of 24 mg/kg per h during the first 28 h following intraperitoneal administration of a 10% ^{14}C-methanol solution (1 g/kg) to male albino rats. By the end of 36 h, 77% of the methanol had been converted to $^{14}CO_2$ and 24% of the dose was excreted unchanged. About equal quantities of methanol were eliminated by the pulmonary and renal plus faecal routes (Tephly et al., 1964).

Comparative studies in rats and monkeys have shown that 75-80% of a 1 g/kg dose of ^{14}C-methanol was recovered as $^{14}CO_2$; 10-18% was excreted unchanged in expired air and 6-11% eliminated in the urine as methanol or formate within a 24-h period (Eells et al., 1981, 1983). Excretion of similar amounts of unchanged methanol eliminated by pulmonary (10-15%) and renal (3-19%) routes in rats and guinea-pigs have also been reported (Bartlett, 1950; Tephly et al., 1964).

After oral administration to dogs of a single dose of methanol (1.97 g/kg), about 10% was excreted unchanged in the urine, over a period of about 100 h. The methanol concentration in the organs was nearly half as high as that found in the urine. About 20% of the administered dose was excreted as formic acid in the urine, which ceased after 100 h. Formic acid concentrations in tissues were about one-half to one-quarter that found in serum (Lund, 1948b).

Oral administration of 2.38 g methanol/kg to male rabbits resulted in 10% of methanol being excreted unchanged in the urine and essentially no increase in formic acid in the urine. Formic acid is oxidized almost completely in the rabbit (Lund, 1948c).

Damian & Raabe (1996) investigated the dose-dependent elimination of formate in male CD rats employing a perfused liver system to separate the kinetic contributions of hepatic metabolism and renal excretion in the total elimination of formate. Formate was eliminated from the perfused rat liver following Michaelis-Menten kinetics. The *in vitro* and *in vivo* dose-dependent studies of formate elimination, in conjunction with the proposed toxicokinetic model (a central, well-mixed compartment and a urine compartment, endogenous production of formate), indicated two main pathways of formate elimination in the rat: (a) hepatic metabolism via Michaelis-Menten kinetics which predominates at low levels, and (b) extremely rapid and extensive urinary excretion that predominates at high dose levels. Urinary excretion consists primarily of glomerular filtration with saturable tubular reabsorption.

6.5 Modelling of pharmacokinetic and toxicokinetic data

Pharmacokinetic and toxicokinetic models have been developed in order to gain better insight into the interspecies variation in the uptake, metabolic fate and excretion of methanol and its metabolites, both compartmentally and physiologically based (Horton et al., 1992; Pollack et al., 1993; Dorman et al., 1994). As has been noted, the elimination of formaldehyde in many species, including primates, is extremely rapid (McMartin et al., 1979).

A pharmacokinetic model of inhaled methanol in humans and comparison to methanol disposition in mice and rats was described by Perkins et al. (1995). Michaelis-Menten elimination parameters (V_{max}= 115 mg/litre per h; k_m = 460 mg/litre) were selected for input into a semi-physiological pharmacokinetic model. Literature values for blood or urine methanol concentrations in humans and non-human primates after methanol inhalation were employed as input to an inhalation disposition model that evaluated the absorption of methanol expressed as the fraction of inhaled methanol concentration that was absorbed. Incorporation of the kinetic parameters and absorption into a pharmacokinetic model of human exposure to methanol, compared to a similar analysis in rodents, indicated that, following an 8-h exposure to 6550 mg/m^3 (5000 ppm) of methanol vapour, blood methanol concentrations in the mouse would be 13-18 fold higher than in humans exposed to the same methanol vapour concentration. Blood methanol concentrations in the rat under similar conditions would be 5-fold higher than in humans. The prediction of higher concentrations in rats was due to the greater respiration rates and consequent greater absorption of methanol by rats.

To address the problems associated with the appropriate design of chronic methanol studies, methanol pharmacokinetics were characterized in male Fischer-344 rats and rhesus monkeys exposed to atmospheric methanol concentrations ranging from 65 to 2600 mg/m^3 (50-2000 ppm) for 6 h (Horton et al., 1992). A physiologically based pharmacokinetic (PBPK) model was then developed to simulate the *in vivo* time course data. The models were used to predict the atmospheric methanol concentration range over which the laboratory species exhibit quantitative similarities with humans. Below 1500 mg/m^3 (1200 ppm) the model predicted all three species would exhibit similar end-of-exposure blood methanol concentrations which would be proportional to atmospheric concentrations. At higher concentrations the increase of methanol in the blood of rats and monkeys was predicted to become non-linear, whereas for humans blood methanol levels were predicted to increase in a linear fashion (Horton et al., 1992).

Female Sprague-Dawley rats at gestational days 7, 14 and 21 and CD-1 mice at gestational days 9 and 18 were exposed to methanol intravenously and orally (100-2500 mg/kg) or by inhalation exposure to 1310 to 26 200 mg/m^3 (1000-20 000 ppm) for 8 h and the concentrations of methanol were measured in blood, urine and amniotic fluid (Pollack & Brouwer, 1996). Methanol disposition was virtually unaffected by pregnancy and the fetal methanol concentrations were approximately similar to those in the mother. Mice accumulated methanol at a rate 2 to 3 times faster than rats, despite the two-fold higher rate of elimination observed in the mouse.

A pharmacokinetic model described the disposition of methanol in rats and mice with the disposition profile being partitioned into saturable and linear metabolic elimination pathways. The saturable pathway was evident at lower doses (100 and 500 mg methanol/kg) and displayed classical carrier-mediated Michaelis-Menten kinetics with a rate-limiting step. The linear pathway, which consisted of passive elimination via pulmonary and urinary clearance of methanol in approximately equal amounts, appeared at the highest dose (2500 mg/kg iv) and displayed the first-order kinetics of elimination that are characteristic of passive-diffusion mechanisms (Pollack & Brouwer, 1996).

In further studies of the comparative toxicokinetics of methanol in pregnant and non-pregnant Sprague-Dawley rats and CD-1 mice (Ward & Pollack, 1996a), methanol disposition in the pregnant rodent was found to be qualitatively similar to that in non-pregnant animals. Rats received a single dose (100 or 2500 mg/kg) of methanol either orally (by gavage) or intravenously; mice received a single oral or intravenous dose of 2500 mg/kg.

The maximal rate of methanol elimination (V_{max}) *in vivo* decreased at term in both species. V_{max} in near-term rats and mice was only 65-80% of that in non-pregnant animals. The kinetic parameters that appeared to be most sensitive to the gestational stage were the rate constants associated with intercompartmental transfer (k_{12} and k_{21}), although there was no obvious relationship between the estimate of these parameters and gestational stage. The data generated in both the *in vivo* and *in vitro* studies demonstrated that alterations in methanol disposition associated with gestational stage should be accounted for in the development of a toxicokinetic model for methanol in pregnant mammals.

The examination of the toxicokinetics of intravenously administered methanol to female Sprague-Dawley rats as a single bolus dose of 50 or 100 mg/kg, or 2500 mg/kg administered over 2 min, resulted in a markedly non-linear elimination of methanol from the systemic circulation suggesting a significant capacity-limited rate of elimination. The data from the 2500 mg/kg group was described by a kinetic model incorporating parallel first-order and saturable elimination processes; a portion of this apparent linear elimination pathway was due to renal excretion of the unchanged alcohol (Pollack et al., 1993). The blood methanol concentration-time profile was consistent with the presence of parallel linear pathways for methanol elimination.

The toxicokinetics of methanol in female CD-1 mice and Sprague-Dawley rats was examined by Ward et al. (1995). Non-linear disposition of methanol was reported in both female CD-1 mice administered a single dose of 2.5 g methanol/kg either by gavage or intravenously (as a 1-min infusion) and Sprague-Dawley rats receiving a single oral dose of 2.5 g/kg. Data obtained after intravenous administration were well-described by a one-compartment model with Michaelis-Menton elimination. Blood methanol concentration-time data after oral administration could be described by a one-compartment (mice) or a two-compartment (rats) model with Michaelis-Menton elimination from the central compartment and biphasic absorption from the gastrointestinal tract. Kinetic parameters (V_{max} for elimination), apparent volume of the central compartment (V_c), first-order rate constants for intercompartmental transfer (k_{12} and k_{21}), and first-order absorption rate constants for fast (k_{AF}) and slow (K_{as}) absorption processes were compared between species. Mice showed a higher maximal elimination rate than rats (when normalized for body weight) ($V_{max} = 117 + 3$ mg/kg per h versus $60.7 + 1.4$ mg/kg per h for rats). Additionally, the contribution of the fast absorption process to overall methanol absorption was larger in the mouse than in the rat. The study demonstrated that the disposition of methanol is similar in rats and mice, although mice eliminated methanol nearly twice as rapidly as rats.

The pharmacokinetics of ^{14}C-methanol and ^{14}C-formate were studied in normal and folate-deficient (FD) female cynomolgus monkeys anaesthetized and exposed by lung-only inhalation to 13, 60, 260 and 1200 mg/m^3 (10, 45, 200 and 900 ppm) ^{14}C-methanol for 2 h to determine the concentration of methanol-derived formate to the total formate pool. The blood concentration of ^{14}C-methanol-derived formate from all exposures was 10-1000 times lower than the endogenous blood formate concentration (0.1-0.2 mmol/litre) reported for monkeys and orders of magnitude lower than levels that produce acute toxicity (8-10 mmol/litre). This suggested that low-level exposure to methanol would not result in elevated blood formate concentrations in humans under short-term exposure conditions (Dorman et al., 1994) (Medkinsky & Dorman, 1985). This was confirmed in a subsequent short-duration inhalation study in which anaesthetized female cynomolgus monkeys were exposed for 2 h to methanol vapour (tagged with radiolabelled carbon) at concentrations of 13, 59, 262 and 1179 mg/m^3 (10, 45, 200 and 900 ppm), and monkeys fed on a diet deficient in folic acid were exposed to

1179 mg/m^3 (900 ppm) for the same duration (Medinsky et al., 1997). The blood levels of methanol increased in a dose-dependent manner. Blood formate levels increased by only a small extent in both groups of monkeys.

7. EFFECTS ON LABORATORY MAMMALS AND *IN VITRO* TEST SYSTEMS

7.1 Single exposure

7.1.1 *Non-primates*

The lethal oral dose of methanol for most experimental animals is relatively high compared to the lethal dose for humans and non-human primates. In all non-primate species that have been studied, methanol has been shown to be the least toxic of the aliphatic alcohols (Koivusalo, 1970). The LD_{50} values or minimum lethal dose for a single oral dose of methanol have been reported to be 9 g/kg for dogs (Gilger & Potts, 1955), 7 g/kg for rabbits (Hunt, 1902; Gilger & Potts, 1955), 7.4-13 g/kg for rats (Gilger & Potts, 1955; Rowe & McCollister, 1982) and 7.3-10 g/kg for mice (Gilger & Potts, 1955; Smith & Taylor, 1982) (Table 4). These doses are 6-10 times the lethal human dose of methanol (Tephly & McMartin, 1984; Jacobsen & McMartin, 1986; HEI, 1987).

Table 4. Single-dose oral toxicity values for methanol in animals

Species	LD_{50} (g/kg)	Reference
Rat	6.2	Kimura et al. (1971)
	9.1	Welch & Slocum (1943)
	9.5 MLD[a]	Gilger & Potts (1955)
	12.9	Deichmann (1948)
	13.0	Smyth et al. (1941)
Mouse	0.420	Smyth et al. (1941)
	7.3-10.0	Smith & Taylor (1982)
Rabbit	7.0 MLD	Gilger & Potts (1955)
Dog	8.0	Gilger & Potts (1955)
Monkey	2-3 MLD	Gilger & Potts (1955)
	7.0 MLD	Cooper & Felig (1961)

[a] Minimum lethal dose

Other reported oral LD_{50} values for methanol in Sprague-Dawley rats varied in 14-day-old, young adult and older rats (7.4, 13.0 and 8.8 ml/kg respectively), suggesting that young adult rats were least susceptible to methanol toxicity (Kimura et al., 1971).

Youssef et al. (1992) reported that the order of oral LD_{50} in adult female albino rats increased as follows: 95/5%-ethanol/methanol, pure methanol, pure ethanol, and 65/35% methanol/ethanol. Clinical features of intoxication in treated rats generally progressed from signs of inebriation to gait disturbances, dose-proportional decreases in response to painful stimuli, respiratory depression and coma, ending in death due to cardio-respiratory failure. In almost all instances, overnight coma was followed by death of the animal. Gross and histopathological examinations of the gastric mucosa revealed diffuse congestion with dilation of gastric blood vessels, but with absence of gross haemorrhage and ulceration.

Rats exposed to 1.0, 2.0 and 3.0 g methanol/kg by gavage exhibited an altered response in an operant conditioning paradigm designed to assess motor deficits produced by neurotoxicants. Methanol decreased the rate of response in a dose-related fashion that suggested impaired coordination and/or reduced endurance (Youssef et al., 1993).

Methanol administered by gavage or intraperitoneally induced hypothermia in Fischer and Long-Evans rats, e.g., brain temperature decreased 1.5 °C within 35 min and colonic temperature was significantly lower (Mohler & Gordon, 1990). This occurred at dose levels of 2-3 g/kg, which is about 20% of the reported LD_{50} value of 10 g/kg in rats (Gilger & Potts, 1955).

Among 40 strains of mice, 72 h oral LD_{50} values ranged from 7.3 to 10.0 g/kg with a mean of 8.68 g/kg methanol for mice fed a standard laboratory chow diet (Smith & Taylor, 1982). Methanol-dosed C57BL/GCs (acatalasemic) mice exhibited slightly lower LD_{50} than Cs^a (normal catalase) mice, irrespective of their folate state (7.1-8.0 versus 8.6-9.0 g/kg). Oral methanol 72-h LD_{50} values ranged from 6.4 to 7.3 kg for mice with folic acid deficiency (FAD) diets, depending upon the concentration of methionine in the diet (0.2-1.8%).

Female minipigs (Minipig YU, Charles River) treated with a single oral dose of methanol at 1, 2.5 and 5.0 g/kg body weight by gavage showed dose-dependent signs of acute methanol intoxication, including mild CNS depression, tremors, ataxia and recumbency, which developed within 0.5-2.0 h and resolved by 52 h. Methanol- and formate-dosed minipigs did not develop optic nerve lesions, toxicologically significant formate accumulation or metabolic acidosis (Dorman et al., 1993).

The effects of single exposures of methanol by inhalation are summarized in Table 5. The following signs of intoxication were noted: increased rate of respiration, a state of nervous depression followed by excitation, irritation of the mucous membranes, loss of weight, ataxia, partial paralysis, prostration, deep narcosis, convulsions and death occurring from respiratory failure (Loewy & von der Heide, 1914; Tyson & Schoenberg, 1914; Eisenberg, 1917; Weese, 1928; Scott et al., 1933; Mashbitz et al., 1936).

Under acute inhalation conditions, folate-deficient Long-Evans male rats exposed to 4000 mg/m^3 (3000 ppm) methanol for 20 h/day did not survive more than 4 days. Rhesus monkeys exposed to 4000 mg/m^3 (3000 ppm) methanol for 21 h/day survived the 20-day exposure period and rhesus monkeys exposed to 13 000 mg/m^3 (10 000 ppm) methanol for 21 h/day survived for more than 4 days (Lee et al., 1994).

The LD$_{50}$ for single intraperitoneal injections of methanol was 10.5-11.0 g/kg in Swiss albino male mice. The animals initially entered into deep narcosis within a few minutes and death usually occurred within 24 h following recovery from deep narcosis (Gilger et al., 1952). The LD$_{50}$ values (mmole/kg) for single intraperitoneal administration were as follows: male Wistar rats, 237; male strain H mice, 336; male Syrian hamster, 267 (Tichy et al., 1985). These values were calculated to correspond to 1489, 1493 and 1499 mmole/m^2 body surface, respectively. Tichy et al. (1985) also determined LD$_{50}$ values for intravenous administration of methanol. The values reported in rats and mice were 66.5 and 147 mmole/kg, corresponding to 418 and 653 mmole/m^2 body surface, respectively.

Studies of rats have indicated that there are changes in levels of dopamine, norepinephrine, serotonin and 5-hydroxyindole acetic acid in various brain regions after a single intraperitoneal injection of

Table 5. Effects from single inhalation exposure to methanol

Animal	Concentration ppm	Duration of exposure (h)	Signs of Intoxication	Outcome	Reference
Mouse	72 600	54	narcosis	died	Weese (1928)
	72 600	28	narcosis	died	
	54 000	54	narcosis	died	
	48 000	24	narcosis	survived	
	10 000	230	ataxia	survived	
	152 800	94 min	narcosis		Mashbitz et al. (1936)
	101 600	91 min	narcosis		
	91 700	95 min	narcosis		
	76 400	89 min	narcosis	overall	
	61 100	134 min	narcosis	mortality	
	45 800	153 min	narcosis	45%	
	30 600	190 min	narcosis		
Rat	60 000	2.5	narcosis convulsions		Loewy & Von Der Heide (1914)
	22 500	8	narcosis		
	13 000	24	prostration		
	8800	8	lethargy		
	4800	8	none		
Dog	3000	8	none		
	32 000	8	prostration incoordination	survived	
	13 700	4	none		
	2000	24	none		

3 g methanol/kg (Jegnathan & Namasivayam, 1989). Studies on the steady-state level of rat brain showed that there was severe depletion of dopamine level in the striatum but a significant increase in the level of dopamine, serotonin and 5-hydroxyindole acetic acid in the hypothalamus. At the same time, norepinephrine and epinephrine levels were reduced in the hypothalamus as well as in the striatum. These effects do not seem to be induced by metabolic acidosis. The changes in monoamine levels are very well correlated with the blood and brain level of methanol as shown by maintaining a higher methanol level either by simultaneous administration of ethanol or by blocking methanol metabolism by pretreatment with 4-methyl pyrazole and 3-amino-1,2,4-triazole. It is thus postulated that monoamine changes induced by methanol appear to be the direct effect of methanol *per se* on the monoaminergic neuronal membranes.

7.1.2 *Non-human primates*

The lethal oral dose of methanol in monkeys (Table 4) has been shown by several investigators to be of the same order of magnitude as the lethal dose for humans. Gilger & Potts (1955) reported a minimum lethal dose (MLD) for methanol of 3 g/kg for the rhesus monkey (*Macaca mulatta*). Clinically the signs of toxicity were similar to those noted in humans. There was a slight initial CNS depression for 1-2 h, followed by a latent period of about 12 h, a progressive weakness, coma and death usually in about 20-30 h. All the monkeys (4) given a lethal dose became severely acidotic within 24 h. Two of the animals showed signs typical of methanol amblyopia observed in humans including dilated, unresponsive pupils and changes of the retina. One monkey exhibited evidence of optic disc hyperaemia and retinal oedema.

Cooper & Felig (1961) reported a MLD dose of 7 g methanol/kg administered orally to rhesus monkeys and observed inebriation, narcosis, coma and death within 24 h (usually without a latent period). Sixteen animals survived 6 g methanol/kg or less. Acidosis (an increased urinary excretion of organic acids) was reported in most cases.

Studies by McMartin et al. (1975) and Clay et al. (1975) were in agreement with earlier studies in monkeys by Gilger & Potts (1955). Rhesus monkeys and pigtail monkeys (*Macaca nemestrina*) administered 3 g methanol/kg orally, showed an initial slight CNS depression followed by a latent period of 12-16 h, during which time the animals showed no obvious signs of toxicity. This was followed by progressive deterioration characterized by anorexia, vomiting, weakness, hyperpnoea and tachypnoea followed by coma with shallow and infrequent respiration and finally death due to respiratory failure 20-30 h after oral administration of methanol. The gradual development of metabolic acidosis coincided with the accumulation of formic acid in the blood and the decrease of bicarbonate in the plasma (McMartin et al., 1975).

An attenuated but prolonged syndrome was produced in monkeys by the administration of an initial methanol dose of 2 g/kg body weight. and subsequent doses (0.5-1.0 g/kg at 12-24 h intervals), producing profound ocular toxicity approximately 40-60 h after the initial dosage (Baumbach et al., 1977; Hayreh et al., 1977; Martin-Amat et al., 1977).

Various species exposed to methanol by inhalation have exhibited haemorrhage, oedema, congestion and pneumonia in the lungs (Eisenberg, 1917; Weese, 1928; Tyson & Schoenberg, 1914). Albuminous and fatty degeneration and fatty infiltration of the liver and kidneys have also been noted (Eisenberg, 1917; Weese, 1928). Fatty degeneration of cardiac muscle has been observed in rabbits exposed repeated over 2 to 6 months to methanol via inhalation (Eisenberg, 1917). This subchronic exposure to methanol in rabbits was also associated with notable central nervous system effects such as optic nerve damage, lesion and atrophy of the cerebrum, cerebellum, medulla and pons, along with decreases in neurocytes, Nissl's granules and in severe cases, parenchyma cells. Repeated inhalation of methanol resulted in hyperaemia of choroid, oedema of ocular tissue including the retina and optic disks, and degeneration of ganglion cells and nerve fibres in a number of species such as the dog, rabbit and monkey (Tyson & Schoenberg, 1914). Acute exposure to methanol via inhalation, as well as oral and dermal exposure, was associated with degeneration and necrosis of parenchymal tissue and neurons, accompanied by capillary congestion and oedema, and degeneration of the retina and optic nerve in rats, rabbits and monkeys (Scott et al, 1933).

An approximate intraperitoneal methanol LD_{50} of 3-4 g/kg for pigtail monkeys (*Macaca nemestrina*) was reported by Clay et al. (1975). Doses of 2 and 3 g/kg produced metabolic acidosis in the animals, while monkeys given 4 g/kg became severely acidotic and exhibited signs of toxicity that were remarkably similar to those reported in human poisoning (Kane et al., 1968). These animals displayed a sharp decrease in blood pH (7.03) at 7.5-21 h after methanol administration. Bicarbonate was the single blood electrolyte observed to change during the course of methanol acidosis. There was a latent period of 15-18 h prior to the onset of overt signs of toxicity, followed by a sequence of signs beginning with behavioural distress, coma within 24-30 h and death. This time-course parallels that reported for humans suffering from methanol poisoning (Röe, 1955).

7.2 Short-term exposure

7.2.1 Inhalation exposure

Male and female Sprague-Dawley rats exposed to 650, 2600 and 6500 mg/m^3 (500, 2000 and 5000 ppm) methanol for 6 h/day, 5 days/week for 4 weeks, exhibited no exposure-related effects except for increased discharges around the nose and eyes which were considered reflective of upper respiratory tract irritation. No consistent treatment-related effects were found for organ weight or body weights or in histopathological or ophthalmoscopical examinations. No ocular effects were noted in rats from 20 repeated exposures to 6500 mg/m^3 (5000 ppm) (Andrews et al., 1987).

Male Sprague-Dawley rats exposed to methanol vapour at concentrations of 260, 2600 and 13 000 mg/m^3 (200, 2000 and 10 000 ppm) for 6 h/day, 5 days/week for 6 weeks, did not develop pulmonary toxicity. No significant changes were found at the lung surface and in lung tissue (White et al., 1983).

Rats exposed to 16.8 methanol (0.022 mg methanol/litre of air) 4 h/day for 6 months and simultaneously administered 0.7 mg methanol/kg daily by gavage exhibited changes in blood morphology, oxidation-reduction processes and liver function (Pavlenko, 1972).

A preliminary study reported that F-344 rats fed control and folate-deficient diets and exposed to methanol at a concentration of 1050 mg/m^3 (800 ppm) for 20 h/day; 7 days/week for 13 weeks showed spontaneous degeneration of retina and optic nerve in both diet groups, while Long-Evans rats did not develop such ocular lesions. The authors suggest that F-344 rats are unsuitable for ocular toxicity studies (Lee et al., 1990).

Mice exposed to 63 000 mg/m^3 (48 000 ppm) methanol for 3.5-4 h/day up to a cumulative total of 24 h were in a state of narcosis but survived, whereas mice became comatose when exposed to 71 000 mg/m^3 (54 000 ppm) for 54 h (Pavlenko, 1972).

Rabbits exposed by inhalation to 61 mg/m^3 (46.6 ppm) methanol for 6 months (duration of exposure/day not reported) exhibited ultrastructural changes in the photoreceptor cells of the retina and Müller fibres (Vendilo et al., 1971).

Two male dogs exposed to methanol vapour in air at 13 000 mg/m^3 (10 000 ppm) for about 3 min in each of 8-h periods/day for 100 consecutive days, exhibited no symptoms, unusual behaviour or visual toxicity. Methanol levels in blood measured at weekly intervals showed median values of 65 and 140 mg/litre blood (Sayers et al., 1944).

In contrast to many studies of methanol toxicity that reported no effect of low doses, two Russian studies (Chao, 1959; Ubaidullaev, 1966) reported evidence of neurobehavioural toxicity at low doses as shown by altered chronaximetry (chronaximetry is the ratio of the minimum time necessary for a stimulus of twice the absolute threshold intensity to evoke a response measured as muscle contractions in response to an electric current applied to an animal's hind leg). Normally, the flexor chronaxia is shorter than the extensor chronaxia, and their ratio is stated to be relatively stable.

Chao (1959) reported that the average chronaxia ratio for rats exposed in the high-dose group (49.77 mg/m^3) for 12 h/day, 5 days/week for 3 months, differed significantly from that in the control group of animals at week 8 of exposure. The average chronaxia ratio returned to normal during the recovery period and the effects in the low-dose group (1.77 mg/m^3) were insignificant. Histopathological changes found in the high-dose group, but not in the low-dose group, included poorly defined changes in the mucous membranes of the trachea and bronchi, hyperplasia of the submucosa of the trachea, slight lymphoid infiltration, swelling and hypertrophy of the muscle layer of arteries, slight degenerative changes to the liver and changes in the neurons of the cerebral cortex (Chao, 1959).

Ubaidullaev (1966) reported that male rats exposed continuously for 90 days to a concentration of 5.3 mg/m³ (4 ppm) of methanol vapour, exhibited changes in chronaxia ratio between antagonistic muscles, in whole blood cholinesterase activity, in urinary excretion of coproporphyrin and in albumin-globulin ratio of the serum. Male rats exposed to 0.57 mg/m³ (0.4 ppm) of methanol vapour continuously for 90 days showed no changes.

It should be noted, however, that an analysis of these studies by Kavet & Nauss (1990) indicated that, due to flaws in the study designs, these studies do not provide adequate evidence of an association between neurobehavioural effects and low-level exposure to methanol. Both studies were limited by the use of small numbers of animals per dose group, as well as insufficient reporting of experimental methods, study results and statistical analysis. Kavet & Nauss (1990) also stated that the biological significance of changes in the chronaxia ratio is uncertain.

Male and female cynomolgus monkeys (*Macaca fascicularis*), three per sex per dose, that were exposed to 650, 2600 and 6500 mg/m³ (500, 2000 and 5000 ppm) methanol for 6 h/day, 5 days/week for 4 weeks showed no upper respiratory tract irritation. Neither gross, microscopic nor ophthalmoscopic examinations disclosed any ocular effects in the monkeys exposed to 6500 mg/m³ (5000 ppm) (Andrews et al., 1987).

7.3   Long-term studies

In two 12-month chronic inhalation studies, Fischer-344 rats (20 female and 20 male animals per group) and B6C3F1 mice (30/30 female/male) were exposed to 13, 130 and 1300 mg/m³ (10, 100 and 1000 ppm) of methanol to examine toxic effects unrelated to carcinogenesis. A concentration of 130 mg/m³ (100 ppm) was found to be the NOEL in both species. At the highest exposure, a slightly reduced weight gain in male and female rats and a small but not significant increase in the relative liver and spleen weight in female rats were observed. In mice, the body weight was significantly higher in the highest exposure groups in both males (after 6 months) and in females (after 9 months). In addition, the incidence and degree of fatty degeneration of hepatocytes was significantly enhanced in the highest exposure groups of mice. However, this could have been due to the higher incidence of fatty degeneration in mice of great body weight. Clinical laboratory results did not show any changes attributable to methanol (NEDO, 1987; Katoh, 1989).

Monkeys (*Macaca fascicularis*) (eight females per group) were exposed to 13, 130 or 1300 mg/m^3 for periods of 22 h/day for up to 29 months. Body weight, haematological and pathological examinations did not reveal any dose-dependent effects except for hyperplasia of reactive astroglias in the nervous system. However, this effect was not correlated to dose or exposure time and was found to be reversible in a recovery test (NEDO, 1982).

7.4 Skin and eye irritation; sensitization

In a modified Magnusson-Kligman maximization test with 10 female guinea-pigs no sensitization was found after intracutaneous or percutaneous induction and challenge with 50% methanol solution in distilled water or with Freud's adjuvant. No skin irritation effects were observed. In a parallel test, a 25% formaldehyde solution was applied in order to test for possible sensitizing effects resulting from the metabolic transformation of methanol to formaldehyde. Again negative test results were seen (BASF, 1979).

New Zealand White albino rabbits treated by application of 100 µl methanol into the lower conjunctival sac according to OECD test guidelines and Draize scoring criteria exhibited the following mean scores of conjunctivitis, chemosis, iritis and corneal opacity after 1, 4, 24, 48 and 72 h (Jacobs, 1990).

Time after application (h):	1	4	24	48	72
Mean score of conjunctivitis:	0.89	2.00	1.67	2.28	2.22
Mean score of chemosis:	2.00	2.00	0.67	1.00	0.50
Mean score of irititis:	0.33	1.00	1.00	0.50	0.33
Mean score of corneal opacity:	0.00	0.00	0.50	0.50	0.67

This demonstrates that methanol causes significant conjunctivitis under the conditions of this test. Initial oedema (chemosis) seen up to 4 h had decreased significantly by 72 h. Other ocular lesions were much less significant.

7.5 Reproductive toxicity, embryotoxicity and teratogenicity

7.5.1 Reproductive toxicity (effects on fertility)

When male Sprague-Dawley rats were exposed for 8 h/day, 5 days/week to airborne methanol concentrations of 260, 2600 or 13 999 mg/m³ (200, 2000 or 10 000 ppm) for 1, 2, 4 or 6 weeks, significantly decreased levels of circulating free testosterone were found among rats exposed to 260 mg/m³ for 2 and 6 weeks and to 2600 mg/m³ for 6 weeks. However, the 13 000 mg/m³ group showed no change. Significant changes in luteinizing hormone (LH) were found after 6 weeks in animals exposed to 13 000 mg/m³, but no changes in follicle-stimulating hormone (FSH) were observed at the various exposure levels (Cameron et al., 1984). Sprague-Dawley rats exposed to 260 mg/m³ for 6 h for either 1 day or 1 week showed significant depression (59%) in serum testosterone immediately after the first exposure, but not after 1 week of daily 6-h exposures (Cameron et al., 1985).

In a subsequent study groups of 10 male Long-Evans hooded rats, 60 days of age and acclimatized (or not) to handling, were exposed to 0, 260, 6500 or 13 000 mg/m³ (0, 200, 5000 or 10 000 ppm) methanol for 6 h and killed either immediately on removal from the chambers or 18 h later. Similar groups of rats, acclimatized to handling or not, were exposed to 6500 mg/m³ during 1, 3 or 6 h and killed immediately. Serum testosterone levels were not significantly increased at 6 or 24 h in acclimatized rats, but levels were increased in non-acclimatized rats exposed to 6500 mg/m³ and killed after 24 h. The serum luteinizing hormone (LH) level was increased in acclimatized rats exposed to 13 500 mg/m³ and killed at 6 and 24 h but the LH level was reduced in non-acclimatized rats exposed to 6500 or 13 000 mg/m³ at 6 h but not 24 h. This experiment did not confirm the earlier report that exposure to 260 mg/m³ for 6 h reduced serum testosterone levels. In the second experiment serum LH and testosterone levels did not differ at any time point between controls and rats exposed to 6500 mg/m³ (Cooper et al.,1992).

Methanol inhalation at 260 mg/m^3 for 8 h/day for up to 6 weeks did not reduce serum testosterone levels in normal Sprague-Dawley rats (Lee et al., 1991). In Long-Evans rats fed either control or folate-reduced diets and exposed to 1040 mg/m^3 for 20 h/day for 13 weeks, no adverse effect on testicular morphology was observed with 10-month-old rats fed either diet. A greater incidence of testicular degeneration was however noted with 18-month-old rats given the folate-reduced diet, suggesting that methanol potentially accelerates the age-related degeneration of the testes (Lee et al., 1991).

7.5.2 *Developmental toxicity*

The inhalation of methanol by pregnant rodents throughout the period of embryogenesis to high atmospheric concentrations (6500 to 26 000 mg/m^3; 5000 to 20 000 ppm) impaired neural tube closure and induced a wide range of concentration-dependent teratogenic and embryolethal effects (Nelson et al., 1985; Rogers et al., 1993; Bolon et al., 1993, 1994). In these studies, significant increase in the incidence of exencephaly were observed following maternal methanol exposures of > 6500 mg/m^3 (> 5000 ppm) in mice, while similar effects were observed in rats following exposures of > 13 000 mg/m^3 (> 10 000 ppm), indicating that mice are more sensitive than rats to the embryotoxic effects of methanol.

Pregnant Sprague-Dawley rats were given by inhalation for 7 h/day either 6500 or 13 000 mg/m^3 (5000, or 10 000 ppm) methanol on days 1-19 of gestation, or 26 000 mg/m^3 (20 000 ppm) methanol on days 7-15 of gestation. The blood levels of methanol in the 26 000 mg/m^3 group ranged from 8.34 to 9.26 mg/ml after 1 day of exposure and from 4.84 to 6.00 mg/ml after 10 days of exposure. Methanol induced a dose-related decrease in fetal weights and an increase in malformations. The highest methanol concentration (26 000 mg/m^3) produced slight maternal toxicity (slightly unsteady gait) after the initial days of exposure, and a high incidence of congenital malformations (p < 0.001), predominantly extra or rudimentary cervical ribs and urinary or cardiovascular defects. Similar malformations were found in the groups exposed to 13 000 mg/m^3 but the incidence was not significantly different from that of the controls. No increase in malformations was found in the group exposed to 6500 mg/m^3 (5000 ppm), which was suggested to be a no-observed-effect level for this test system (Nelson et al., 1985).

Pregnant CD-1 mice were treated by inhalation to 1300, 2600, 6500, 10 000, 13 000 or 19 500 mg/m³ (1000, 2000, 5000, 7500, 10 000 or 15 000 ppm) of methanol for 7 h/day on days 6-15 of pregnancy. Significant increases were observed in the incidence of exencephaly and cleft palate at 6500 mg/m³ or more. Increased embryo/fetal death was found at exposures of 10 000 mg/m³ or more, including an increasing incidence of full-litter resorptions. Reduced fetal weight was found at 13 000 mg/m³ or more. A dose-related increase in cervical vertebrae was significant at 2600 mg/m³ or more. The NOAEL for the developmental toxicity was suggested to be 1300 mg/m³ (1000 ppm) methanol in this test system. There was no evidence of maternal toxicity at methanol exposures below 10 000 mg/m³ (Rogers et al., 1993).

A spectrum of cephalic neural tube defects was found in near-term (gestation day 17) CD-1 mouse fetuses following maternal inhalation of methanol at high concentration (19 500 mg/m³; 15 000 ppm) for 6 h/day during neurulation (gestation days 7-9). Dysraphism, chiefly exencephaly, occurred in 15% of the fetuses, usually in association with reduction or absence of multiple bones in the craniofacial skeleton and ocular anomalies (prematurely open eyelids, cataracts, retinal folds). Exposure to a high concentration of methanol (19 500 mg/m³) injured the multiple stem populations in the neuralating mouse embryo. Significant neural pathology may remain in older conceptuses even in the absence of gross lesions (Bolon et al., 1994).

Transient neurological signs and reduced body weights were found in up to 20% of CD-1 dams exposed to 19 500 mg/m³ (15 000 ppm) methanol 6 h/day throughout organogenesis (gestational days 6-15). Near-term fetuses revealed embryotoxicity (increased resorptions, reduced fetal weights and/or fetal malformations) at 13 000 and 19 500 mg/m³ (10 000 and 15 000 ppm) methanol while 3-day exposures at 6500 mg/m³ (5000 ppm) for 6 h/day yielded no observable adverse effects (Bolan et al., 1993). In the studies of Bolon et al. (1993, 1994), terata included neural and ocular defects, cleft palate, hydronephrosis, deformed tails and limb (paw and digit) anomalies. Neural tube defects and ocular lesions occurred after methanol inhalation by pregnant CD-1 mice between gestational days 7 and 9, while limb anomalies were induced only during gestational days 9-11; cleft palate and hydronephrosis were observed after exposure during either period. The spectrum of teratogenic effects depended upon both the stage of embryonic development and the number of methanol exposures.

Long-Evans rats administered single oral doses of 1.3, 2.6 or 5.2 ml methanol/kg by gavage on day 10 of gestation, exhibited dose-related anomalies, e.g., undescended testes and eye defects (exophthalmia and anophthalmia) in the offspring. At the methanol dose of 5.2 ml/kg, the maternal weight loss was > 10%, which was the only clinical toxic manifestation/histopathological change noted for the dams. A significant decrease in fetal body weight (11-21%) was associated with oral ingestion of methanol in the dams. Methanol given acutely can produce anomalies in the offspring where there are no apparent maternal toxic responses (Youssef et al., 1991).

Methanol was shown to impair uterine decidualization during early pregnancy in Holtzman rats administered 1.6, 2.4 or 3.2 g methanol/kg per day by gavage during days 1-8. Reductions in pregnant uterine and implantation site weights seen on day 9 were the result of methanol impedance of normal uterine decidualization as demonstrated by effects on decidual cell response technique. Methanol (3.2 g/kg per day) produced a non-specific maternal toxicity (reduction in body weight) by day 9, but no effect on days 11 or 20 on embryo and fetal survival or development were found (Cummings, 1993).

When pregnant CD-1 mice were gavaged orally with 4 g methanol/kg, the incidences of fetal resorption, external defects (including cleft palate) and reduced fetal weight were similar to those observed in the 13 000 mg/m^3 (10 000 ppm) inhalation exposure group. Cleft palate (43.5% per litter) and exencephaly (29% per litter) were the predominant external defects seen following methanol exposure by oral gavage. Methanol blood level in the gavage study was 4 mg/ml, which was reportedly similar to the blood level at the 13 000 mg/m^3 inhalation exposure group (see above) (Rogers et al., 1993).

No effects on reproductive performance were reported in a two-generation reproductive study in F-344 rats administered 13, 130 or 1300 mg/m^3 (10, 100 or 1000 ppm) methanol by inhalation for 18-20 h/day. A statistically significant decrease in brain weight was found at the 1300 mg/m^3 level in 3-, 6- and 8-week-old pups of the F_1 generation. In the F_2 generation reduced brain thymus and hypophysis weight was observed. (NEDO, 1987; Katoh, 1989).

Teratology studies with Sprague-Dawley rats exposed to 260, 1300 or 6500 mg/m³ (200, 1000 or 5000 ppm) methanol by inhalation for 22 h/day during gestational days 7-17 revealed significant weight decreases in brain, thyroid and thymus of the offspring resulting from maternal exposure to 6500 mg/m³. However, no abnormal changes were detected histopathologically. Evidence of maternal toxicity was found at this level of exposure and toxic effects to fetuses were reported, including death. No effects were found at 1300 kg/m³ (NEDO, 1987; Katoh, 1989).

A pilot developmental toxicity study was conducted by Ryan et al. (1994) to assess the utility of the folic-acid-deficient rat model, a model that would be sensitive to methanol and potentially reflective of the human risk/response. Methanol was administered in drinking-water on days 6-15 of gestation at concentrations of 0.5, 1.0 and 2.0% to three groups of 7 to 9 sperm-positive Long-Evans rats. The average blood levels were given as 0.21, 0.26 and 0.67 mg/ml, respectively. A dose-dependant increase in the incidence of maternal and developmental effects was observed. For both end-points the NOEL was assumed to be less than 0.5% methanol in drinking-water, corresponding to a blood level of 0.21 mg/ml.

Weiss et al. (1996) studied developmental neurotoxicity of pregnant Long-Evans rats and their newborn offspring exposed to 5900 mg/m³ (4500 ppm) of methanol by inhalation for 6 h daily, beginning on gestation day 6, with both dams and pups then being exposed through postnatal day 21. Although findings suggested significant functional consequences in rats resulting from this exposure, these consequences were considered subtle in character. Exposure to 5900 mg methanol/m³ did not affect the suckling time and conditioned olfactory aversion test of newborn rats. Methanol-exposed newborn pups were less active on postnatal day 18 and more active on postnatal day 25 than control newborn pups (motor activity test). The study found only isolated positive results that were small and variable. The two adult assays, the fixed-ratio wheel-running test and the stochastic discrimination test, yielded evidence of a significant methanol effect.

No evidence of brain damage emerged on the basis of neuropathology, although differences in neural cell adhesion molecules (NCAMs) arising from methanol exposure were observed in neonatal cerebella (Weiss et al., 1996). Methanol treatment caused a decrease in expression in both NCAM 140 and NCAM 180.

Further elaboration of the effects of perinatal exposure on NCAM in Long-Evans rats exposed to 5900 mg/m^3 (4500 ppm) methanol vapour for 6 h daily (beginning on gestation day 6 with dams and pups then exposed until postnatal day 21) were described by Stern et al. (1996). Blood methanol concentrations from samples obtained immediately following a 6-h exposure reached approximately 500-800 µg/ml in the dams during gestation, and lactation average concentrations for pups attained levels about twice those of the dams. Light-microscopic analysis showed no significant abnormalities in the brains of the methanol-treated animals. However, assays of NCAM in the brains of pups sacrificed on postnatal day 4 showed staining for both the 140 and the 180 kDa isoforms to be less intense in the cerebellum of exposed animals. NCAM differences were not apparent in animals sacrificed after their final exposure. NCAM 140 is the primary isoform expressed during the stages of neuronal migration and NCAM 180 is expressed during synaptogenesis where it is critical to neuronal plasticity, learning and memory. NCAMs are developmentally regulated glycoproteins that serve critical roles in the formation and maintenance of the nervous system (Stern et al., 1996).

7.5.3 Behavioural effects

Neonatal behavioural toxicity was reported in studies involving two groups of primigravid Long-Evans rats given drinking solutions of 2% methanol either on gestational days 15-17 or 17-19, with the average daily intake on these days amounting to 2.5 g methanol/kg. Lack of maternal toxicity was indicated by measurements of weight gain, gestational duration or daily fluid intake. Litter size, birth weight and infant mortality did not differ between the two treatment groups and the control. Pups from methanol-treated rats required longer periods than controls to begin suckling on postnatal day 1. On postnatal day 10, they required more time to locate nesting material from their home cages, suggesting that prenatal methanol exposure induced behavioural abnormalities early in life, unaccompanied by overt toxicity (Infurna & Weiss, 1986).

Following inhalation exposure of Long-Evans rats to 19 500 mg/m^3 (15 000 ppm) methanol for 7 h/day on gestational days 7-19, maternal blood levels decreased significantly from 3.8 mg/litre on the first day of exposure to 3.1 mg/litre on the 12th day of exposure. Methanol transiently reduced maternal body weight by 4-7% on gestational days 8-10 and offspring body weight by 5% on post-natal days 1-3. Motor activity, olfactory learning, behavioural thermoregulation, T-maze learning, acoustic startle response, pubertal landmarks and passive avoidance tests performed at the end of the exposure period failed to reveal significant effects. Prenatal exposure to high levels of inhaled methanol appeared to have little effect beyond post-natal day 3 in this series of tests (Stanton et al., 1995).

7.5.4   *In vitro studies*

Methanol is developmentally toxic to both mouse (CD-1) and rat (Sprague-Dawley) embryos during organogenesis in whole embryo culture (WEC), a technique which removes the confounding maternal influences (Andrews et al., 1993). Comparable developmental stages of CD-1 mouse and Sprague-Dawley rat embryos were exposed to methanol (0-16 mg/ml for rat and 0-8 mg/ml for mouse embryos) for 24 h. Rat embryos were cultured for an additional 24 h without methanol in the medium, having a total culture time of 48 h. Concentration-dependent decreases in somite number, head length and developmental score occurred in both species, with significant effects in the rat at ≥ 8 mg/ml and in the mouse at ≥ 4 mg/ml (Andrews et al., 1993).

In studies of 8-day mouse embryos cultured in methanol, concentrations greater than 2 mg methanol/ml caused a significant decrease in developmental score and crown-rump length; the 8 mg/ml group also suffered 80% embryolethality (Andrews et al., 1993). Mouse embryos were affected at methanol concentrations that were not dysmorphogenic or embryotoxic in the rat following teratogenic *in vivo* exposures (Rogers et al, 1993), suggesting that the higher sensitivity of the mouse was due, at least in part, to the greater intrinsic embryonal sensitivity of this species to methanol (Andrews et al., 1993).

Depending on the concentration and duration of methanol exposure (0-20 mg/ml for 6 h, 12 h, or 1 or 4 days) on embryonic CD-1 mouse palate in serum-free organ culture, the medial epithelium either degenerated completely or remained intact in unfused palates (either condition would interfere with fusion) (Abbott et al., 1994). Cellular proliferation appeared to be a specific and sensitive target for methanol as craniofacial tissues responded to methanol with reduction in DNA content at an exposure that did not effect total protein. However both DNA and protein levels decreased with increasing exposure to methanol. Methanol selectively altered the morphological fate of the medial palatal epithelium cells and the specific effect on cell survival was exposure dependent (Abbott et al., 1994).

7.6 Mutagenicity and related end-points

7.6.1 In vitro studies

The structure of methanol (by analogy with ethanol) does not suggest that it would be genotoxic.

Methanol gave negative results when tested in *Salmonella typhimurium* plate incorporation assays with or without metabolic activation using strains TA98, TA100, TA1535, TA1537 and TA1538 (Simmon et al., 1977). It was also negative in the presence or absence of metabolic activation in strains TA1535, TA100, TA1538, TA98 and TA1537 (De Flora et al., 1984) and in a DNA repair test in *E. coli* using strains WP 2, WP 67 and CM 871 in the presence or absence of metabolic activation (De Flora et al., 1984).

Methanol (6.0% v/v) induced 3.02% chromosomal malsegregation in *Aspergillus nidulans* diploid strain P1 (Crebelli et al., 1989). The result was statistically significant at two concentrations and a dose-response relationship was evident.

Methanol was negative for gene mutation at the ade 6 locus in the yeast *Schizosaccharomyces pombe* with or without the postmitochondrial fraction from mouse liver (Abbondandolo et al., 1980). It was also negative in a mutagenicity test for n+1 aneuploidy arising from meiotic disfunction of linkage group I in the fungus *Neurospora crassa* (Griffiths, 1981).

Methanol did not induce sister chromatid exchanges (SCEs) in Chinese hamster cells *in vitro* during treatment for 8 days to a final concentration of 0.1% (v/v) (Obe & Ristow, 1977). Only in the presence of S-9 mix and methanol (7.9 mg/ml) was there a significant increase in the mutation frequency in L5178Y mouse lymphoma cells (McGregor et al., 1985), possibly because this assay detects chromosome damage as well as gene mutation.

Methanol was negative in two *in vitro* tests for cell transformation: the Syrian hamster embryo cell (SHE) clonal system (Pienta et al., 1977) and the Rausher leukaemia virus-infected rat embryo cell (RLV/RE system) (Heidelberger et al., 1983).

Addition of methanol (or ethanol) to unleaded gasoline as a fuel extender did not appear to significantly alter the genetic toxicity of particulate exhaust particles when tested in *S. typhimurium* strains TA100, TA98, TA98 NR, and TA98 DNPR with S-9 activation. In all the alcohol-blended fuel tests, the mass of particle-associated organics emitted from the exhaust was lower than that observed during the control tests using gasoline alone (Clark et al., 1983).

7.6.2 *In vivo studies*

No increased frequencies of micronuclei in blood cells, of SCEs, chromosome aberrations or micronuclei in lung cells, or of synaptonemal complex damage in spermatocytes were found in mice exposed by inhalation to 1050 or 5200 mg/m^3 (800 or 4000 ppm) methanol for 5 days (Campbell et al., 1991).

Urine from mice orally administered five daily doses of methanol (5 g/kg total) showed no mutagenic activity, and no increase in the incidence of abnormal sperm was reported (Chang et al., 1983). Oral administration of 1 g methanol/kg to mice increased the incidence of chromosomal aberrations, particularly aneuploidy and SCEs, as well as the incidence of micronuclei in polychromatic erythrocytes (Pereira et al., 1982).

The oral administration of ^{14}C-labelled methanol to rats resulted in covalent binding to haemoglobin, with binding exhibiting a linear dose relationship between 10 and 100 μmol/kg (Pereira et al., 1982).

B6C3F$_1$ mice treated with five daily oral doses of 1 g methanol/kg exhibited abnormal (banana type) sperm morphology. The biological significance of these changes is unknown (Ward et al., 1984). It should be noted that the above results, namely altered sperm (Ward et al., 1984) and haemoglobin binding (Pereira et al., 1982) are end-points not generally used for genotoxic evaluation and their assessment in terms of mutagenicity is unclear.

There is some evidence that bone marrow cytogenetic analysis indicated a dose-related response for structural aberrations, especially centric fusions in mice treated with three daily intraperitoneal methanol doses of between 75-300 mg/kg total dose (Chang et al., 1983).

In vitro and *in vivo* mutagenicity studies on methanol, i.e., the Ames test, somatic mutation assay in CH-V79 cells, chromosome aberrations, SCEs and the micronucleus test in mice conducted by NEDO (1987; Katoh, 1989), were all reported to be negative.

7.7 Carcinogenicity

There have been no studies reported in the peer-reviewed literature on the potential carcinogenicity of methanol *per se* in laboratory animals.

The New Energy Development Organization (NEDO) in Japan reported carcinogenicity studies in which B6C3F$_1$ mice and Fischer-344 rats of both sexes were exposed by inhalation to 13, 130 or 1300 mg/m^3 (10, 100 and 1000 ppm) methanol for 20 h/day for 18 and 24 months, respectively (NEDO, 1987; Katoh, 1989). No evidence of carcinogenicity was found in either species. High-dosed animals had a higher, but not statistically significant, incidence of papillary adenomas than controls , and histopathological examination suggested that these changes were between non-neoplastic and neoplastic changes. Additionally, seven cases of adrenal pheochromocytoma were found in high-dose animals compared to one case in controls. This observation was not statistically significant according to the Fisher exact test (Katoh, 1989).

It is unlikely that methanol is carcinogenic to mouse skin. In an experiment using four strains of female mice (Balb/c, Sencar, CD-1 and Swiss) to study *N*-nitrosomethylurea carcinogenesis, methanol was used as a solvent control. Four groups of 20 mice of each strain received 25 µl methanol twice weekly for 50 weeks followed by observation for lifespan. Only one skin tumour was observed among the 80 control animals (Lijinsky et al., 1991).

7.8 Special studies

7.8.1 *Effects on hepatocytes*

When Garcia & Van Zandt (1969) administered repeated doses of 3 to 6 g/kg by gavage to rhesus monkeys (*Macaca mulata*) for 3-20 weeks, average serum levels of methanol of 4750 mg/litre were attained within a few hours. Animals were killed at the end of treatment and livers examined histologically. Hepatocytes showed nucleolar segregation (zoning of nucleus), hyperplasia of endoplasmic reticulum and swelling of mitochondria. These changes were also found in one monkey sacrificed 12 weeks after the end of treatment.

7.8.2 *Toxic interactions*

Inhaled methanol potentiated the hepatotoxicity produced by carbon tetrachloride in adult male F-344 rats. Rats were exposed to methanol (0 or 13 000 mg/m^3) 10000 ppm for 6 h, then treated 24 h later with oral CCl_4 (0.075 ml/kg). CCl_4 alone produced a low level of hepatotoxicity within 3 days. Methanol plus CCl_4 resulted in marked increases in serum aspartate aminotransferase and alanine amino-transferase that lasted for 7 days. Methanol also exacerbated the histological evidence of CCl_4-induced centrilobular degeneration and necrosis (Simmons et al., 1995).

Methanol exposure by inhalation induced cytochrome P4502E1 (CYP2E1), which appeared to be the principal toxicokinetic mechanism underlying methanol potentiation of carbon tetrachloride hepatotoxicity (Allis et al., 1996).

When dichloromethane (DCM) is metabolized carbon monoxide is formed, leading to increased carboxyhaemoglobin (COHb) levels in blood. Pankow & Jagielki (1993) found that in rats pretreated with methanol, methanol doses of 790-6330 mg/kg (24.7-198 mmol/kg) stimulated increased metabolism of DCM, as seen by further increases in COHb levels. When methanol was administered simultaneously with DCM, a decrease in COHb formation was seen at methanol doses of 4736 to 7900 mg/kg (148-247 mmol/kg) but not at 3162 mg/kg (98.8 mmol/kg). Thus methanol can interact with DCM metabolism both by induction and by competitive inhibition, the latter only at very high doses.

Poon et al. (1994) reported no significant interactive effects in young Sprague-Dawley rats exposed to vapours of methanol/toluene (400/110 mg/m^3; 400/1100 mg/m^3; 4000/110 mg/m^3 and 4000/1100 mg/m^3) for 6 h/day, 5 days/week for 4 weeks. Exposure to methanol (400 to 4000 mg/m^3) and to toluene (110 mg/m^3 to 1100 mg/m^3) or to a mixture of both produced mild biochemical effects and histological changes in the thyroid (moderate reduction in follicle size in the thyroids) and nasal passages.

The biochemical, haematological and histological effects on Sprague-Dawley rats after exposure to methanol (3000 mg/m^3; 2500 ppm), gasoline (3200 ppm) and methanol/gasoline (2500/3200 ppm) vapour 6 h/day for 4 weeks were examined by Poon et al. (1995). Gasoline was largely responsible for the adverse effects, the most significant of which included depression in weight gain in the males, increased liver weight and hepatic microsomal enzyme activities in both sexes, and suppression of uterine eosinophilia. No apparent interactive effects between methanol and gasoline were observed.

7.8.3 Studies with exhaust emissions from methanol-fuelled engines

There are few data related to the effects of emissions from methanol-fuelled engines. Since most such fuels will contain a proportion of gasoline and other additives and the emissions will be complex, the interpretation of these data in relation to methanol toxicity is complicated.

Maejima et al. (1992, 1993 and 1994) studied the effects of emissions from M-85 methanol-fuelled engines (methanol with 15% gasoline), without a catalyst, on Fischer-344 rats for periods up to 12 weeks. The exhaust contained significant amounts of carbon monoxide (89.9 ppm), oxides of nitrogen (22.9 ppm), formaldehyde (2.3 ppm) and methanol (8.1 ppm). The effects observed were considered to be primarily related to formaldehyde. No increase in plasma methanol or formic acid was detected.

7.9 Mechanism of ocular toxicity

Formic acid, the toxic metabolite of methanol, has been hypothesized to produce retinal and optic nerve toxicity by disrupting mitochondrial energy production (Fig. 1) (Martin-Amat et al., 1977; Sharpe et al., 1982). It has been shown *in vitro* to inhibit the activity of cytochrome oxidase, a vital component of the mitochondrial electron transport chain involved in ATP synthesis (Nicholls, 1975). Inhibition occurs subsequent to the binding of formic acid to the ferric haem iron of cytochrome oxidase, and the apparent inhibition constant is between 5 and 30 mM (Nicholls, 1975). Concentrations of formate present in the blood and tissues of methanol-intoxicated humans, non-human primates and rodent models of methanol-intoxication are within this range (Martin-Amat et al., 1977; Sejersted et al., 1983; Eells, 1991).

Studies conducted in methanol-sensitive rodent models have revealed abnormalities in retinal and optic nerve function and morphology, consistent with the hypothesis that formate acts as a mitochondrial toxin (Fig. 2). In these animal models, formate oxidation is selectively inhibited by dietary (Lee et al., 1994) or chemical (Eells et al., 1981) depletion of folate coenzymes, thus allowing formate to accumulate to toxic concentrations following methanol administration. Methanol-intoxicated rats developed formic acidaemia, metabolic acidosis and visual toxicity analogous to the human methanol poisoning syndrome (Eells, 1991; Murray et al., 1991; Lee et al., 1994a,b).

Sixty hours after the administration of the first dose of methanol, blood formate values ranged from 8-20 mM with blood hydrogen carbonate values in the range of 5-12 mEq/litre and blood pH values of 6.83-7.08. Similar blood formate concentrations, hydrogen carbonate levels and pH values were reported in methanol-intoxicated monkeys (Martin-Amat et al., 1977) and in severe cases of human methanol poisoning (McMartin et al., 1980a; Sejersted et al., 1983; Jacobsen et al., 1988).

Visual dysfunction was measured as reduction in the flash evoked cortical potential (FEP) and electroretinogram (ERG). The FEP is a measure of the functional integrity of the primary visual pathway from the retina to the visual cortex and the ERG is a global measure of retinal function in response to illumination (Creel et al., 1970; Dowling, 1987). The FEP was progressively diminished in methanol-intoxicated rats, indicative of a disruption of neuronal conduction along the primary visual pathway from the retina to the visual cortex (Eells, 1991). ERG analysis in methanol-intoxicated rats revealed a significant early deficit in *b*-wave amplitude, followed by a temporally delayed lesser reduction in *a*-wave amplitude (Murray et al., 1991).

The *b*-wave of the ERG is generated by depolarization of the Muller glial cells and reflects synaptic activity at the level of the bipolar cells (Dowling, 1987). The *b*-wave of the ERG is extremely sensitive to conditions that interfere with retinal energy metabolism and is reduced or abolished following brief ischaemia or the administration of metabolic poisons (Bresnick, 1989; Dowling, 1987). Both FEP and ERG alterations occurred at the same time as accumulation of blood formate, indicative of a causal relationship between formate-induced metabolic and visual disturbances. Similar ERG reductions have been reported in methanol-intoxicated primates (Ingemansson, 1983) and in human methanol intoxication (Ruedemann, 1962; Murray et al., 1991).

In addition to neurofunctional changes, bioenergetic and morphological alterations indicative of formate-induced disruption of retinal energy metabolism have been documented in methanol-intoxicated rats (Murray et al., 1991; Eells et al., 1996; Garner et al., 1995a,b). Morphological studies, coupled with cytochrome oxidase histochemistry, revealed generalized retinal oedema, photoreceptor and RPE vacuolation, mitochondrial swelling and a reduction in cytochrome oxidase activity in photoreceptor mitochondria from methanol-intoxicated rats (Murray et al., 1991; Eells et al., 1995, 1996). The most striking structural alterations observed in the retinas of methanol-intoxicated rats were vacuolation and mitochondrial swelling in inner segments of the photoreceptor cells (Murray et al., 1991). Photoreceptor mitochondria from methanol-intoxicated rats were swollen and expanded to disrupted cristae and showed no evidence of cytochrome oxidase reaction product. In contrast, photoreceptor mitochondria from control animals showed normal morphology with well-defined cristae and were moderately reactive for cytochrome oxidase reaction product. These findings are consistent with disruption of ionic homoeostasis in the photoreceptors, secondary to inhibition of mitochondrial function. Biochemical measurements also showed a significant reduction in retinal and brain cytochrome oxidase activity and ATP concentrations in methanol-intoxicated rats relative to control animals (Eells et al., 1995). Surprisingly, no differences from control values were observed in hepatic, renal or cardiac cytochrome oxidase activity or ATP concentrations in methanol-intoxicated rats. The reduction in retinal function, inhibition of retinal, optic nerve and brain cytochrome oxidase activity, depletion of retinal and brain ATP concentrations, and mitochondrial disruption produced in methanol-intoxicated rats are consistent with the hypothesis that formate acts as a mitochondrial toxin with selectivity for the retina and brain.

Studies by Eells et al. (1996) compared the effects on retinal function and structure of rapidly increasing formate concentrations typical of acute methanol intoxication with low-level plateau formate concentrations more likely to be generated by subacute or chronic methanol exposure. Methanol-intoxicated rats that accumulated formate concentrations of 8-15 mM developed metabolic acidosis, retinal dysfunction, and retinal histopathological changes. Retinal dysfunction was measured as reductions in the *a*- and *b*-waves of the electroretinogram that occurred at the same time as blood formate accumulation. Histopathological studies revealed vacuolation in the retinal pigment epithelium and photoreceptor inner segments. Rats exposed to formate concentrations ranging from 4 to 6 mM for 48 h showed evidence of retinal dysfunction in the absence of metabolic acidosis and retinal histopathology. These data indicated that formate-induced retinal dysfunction in methanol-intoxicated rats can be produced by steadily increasing concentrations of formate and, importantly, can also be produced by prolonged exposure to lower concentrations of formate.

Martinasevic et al. (1996) studied components of folate-dependent formate oxidation, e.g., folate and 10-CHO-H$_4$-folate dehydrogenase (10-FDH), in human and rat retinae. Total folate levels in human and rat retinal tissues were much lower than the levels in liver. However, folate levels in human retina were only 14% of those determined in rat retina. Comparable amounts of this 10-FDH were present in both cellular compartments in each species. However, the amount of 10-FDH in the human retina was approximately three times the amount found in the rat retina. Immunohistochemical staining for 10-FDH showed that this enzyme was preferentially localized in Müller cells. Since Müller cells appear to represent the target for formate-induced ocular toxicity, the authors suggested that formate oxidation reactions might serve two roles, first a protective role and then a role in methanol-induced toxicity in Müller cells.

Garner & Lee (1994) employing oscillatory potential analysis showed that retinal ischaemia was not involved in methanol-induced visual system toxicity.

The role of retinal metabolism in methanol-induced retinal toxicity in folate-sufficient (FS) rats and folate-deficient (FR) rats, some of which were also pretreated with disulfiram (DSF), was examined by Garner et al. (1995). Folate-deficient rats treated with methanol displayed elevated blood and vitreous humour formate levels along with abnormal electroretinograms (ERG), whereas methanol-exposed folate-deficient rats pretreated with DSF did not. Formaldehyde was not detected in blood or vitreous humour, either with or without DSF treatment, suggesting that formate is the toxic metabolite in methanol-induced retinal toxicity. Additionally, intravenous infusion of formate to levels seen in methanol toxicity did not alter ERG levels, suggesting intraretinal metabolism of methanol to formate may be necessary for retinal toxicity.

Studies measuring ATP synthesis in mitochondria isolated from bovine retina and bovine heart have provided additional evidence for a tissue-selective action of formate (Eells et al., in press). In these studies, mitochondrial ATP synthesis was measured in the presence of different metabolic substrates. Formate selectively inhibited ATP synthesis in mitochondria isolated from bovine retina in the presence of metabolic substrates supplying electrons at the level of complex I, complex II and complex IV in the mitochondrial respiratory chain. The inhibitory effect of formate on retinal mitochondrial ATP synthesis was concentration-dependent, significant reductions in ATP synthesis being produced at 10 mM formate and K_i values for inhibition ranging from 30 to 50 mM formate. Comparative studies conducted in mitochondria isolated from bovine heart showed little or no inhibition of ATP synthesis at formate concentrations up to 50 mM. These findings provide direct evidence that formate acts as retinal mitochondrial toxin and suggest that one component of the retinotoxic actions of formate may be due to tissue-specific differences in mitochondrial transport mechanisms or in mitochondrial metabolism.

The apparent selective vulnerability of the retina and optic nerve to the toxic actions of formate in methanol poisoning has been the subject of considerable speculation (Röe, 1955; Sharpe et al., 1982; Jacobsen & McMartin, 1986). Although methanol intoxication is known to disrupt brain function and severe intoxication results in coma and death, the most common permanent consequence of methanol intoxication is blindness (Röe, 1955). Several factors may contribute to the unique vulnerability of the retina and optic nerve to the cytotoxic actions of formate. One component of this selectivity is related to the differences in the distribution of formate in the eye and the brain. Formate concentrations measured in the vitreous humour and retinas of methanol-intoxicated rats (Eells, 1991; Eells et al., 1996) were equivalent to or greater than corresponding blood formate concentrations. In contrast, the concentrations of formate in the brain were significantly lower than blood formate concentrations. These data suggest that the toxic actions of methanol on the visual system may be due to the selective accumulation of formate in the vitreous humour and the retina as compared with other regions of the central nervous system. Secondly, the retina has a very limited metabolic capacity to oxidize and thus detoxify formate (Eells et al., 1996). Thirdly, cytochrome oxidase activity and ATP concentrations have been shown to be selectively reduced in the retina, optic nerve and brain in methanol-intoxicated rats, suggesting that there may be tissue- and cell-specific differences in mitochondrial populations and in the actions of formate on mitochondrial function (Eells et al., 1995). Finally, *in vitro* studies in isolated retinal and cardiac mitochondria have shown that formate selectively inhibits retinal mitochondrial ATP synthesis (Eells et al., in press). These findings support the hypothesis that formate acts as a selective mitochondrial toxin in the retina and establish a link between the effects of formate *in vitro* and the retinal toxicity associated with formate accumulation in methanol intoxication.

8. EFFECTS ON HUMANS

Acute oral and inhalation exposures, and to a lesser extent percutaneous absorption of high concentrations of methanol, have resulted in CNS depression, blindness, coma and death. The most noted effects resulting from longer-term exposure to lower levels of methanol have been a broad range of ocular effects.

8.1 General population and occupational exposure

The human health effects after exposure to methanol are qualitatively the same for the general population and for those exposed in the workplace, and will be considered together. Acute methanol intoxication in the general population is an uncommon occurrence, but often results in serious morbidity and mortality. Litovitz et al. (1988) reviewed the acute methanol exposure cases reported in the USA. In 1987, 1601 methanol poisonings were reported to the American Association of Poison Control Centers (AAPCC). Half of these individuals required hospitalization and the death rate was 0.375%. It was estimated that the actual annual incidence of methanol poisonings in the USA in 1987 was about 6400 cases. Subsequent surveys of methanol exposure cases have been conducted by the AAPCC, and these have shown similar annual frequencies to that in 1987. These data result from poisoning cases that are not usually reported elsewhere, since case reports of methanol poisoning are rarely published in today's literature. Poisoning frequency surveys are not available from the rest of the world, but reports in the biomedical literature and in the press would suggest a worldwide distribution of methanol poisoning cases at least as great as in the USA.

8.1.1 Acute toxicity

Methanol (wood alcohol) has been recognized as a human toxic agent since the end of the 19th century. Since the early part of the 20th century, many hundreds of cases of methanol intoxication have been reported as single cases and as groups in many countries. Many of the human cases were due to the ingestion of denatured alcohol.

The preponderance of methanol poisonings have resulted from the consumption of adulterated alcoholic beverages, e.g., "moonshine", or "bootleg whiskey", wood alcohol and spirits mixed with whiskey. Buller & Wood (1904) and Wood & Buller (1904) reported 235 cases of blindness or death primarily connected with drinking adulterated beverages or wood alcohol products, but these also included 10 deaths involving inhalation or absorption of methanol through the skin.

Bennett et al. (1953) described a case that occurred in Atlanta, Georgia, USA, in 1951, when within a 5-day period, 323 people consumed bootlegged whiskey contaminated with 35-40% methanol and 41 of them died. Kane et al. (1968) reported the poisoning of 18 individuals, of whom 8 died, when a diluted paint thinner containing approximately 37% (by volume) methanol was used as an alcoholic beverage in Lexington, Kentucky, USA.

An epidemic in the State Prison of Southern Michigan in 1979 in which methanol diluent used in photocopying machines was used as "home-made" spirits (containing approximately 3% methanol) resulted in 46 definite cases of methanol intoxication and 3 deaths (Swartz et al., 1981). Methanol poisoning among 23 servicemen in an Army hospital in Korea who had ingested bootleg sake contaminated with methanol was reported by Keeney & Mellinkoff (1951). Tonning et al. (1956) reported acute methanol poisoning in 49 naval personnel who consumed drinks made from duplicating fluid containing a high concentration of methanol.

An outbreak of acute methanol intoxication involving 28 young men in Papua New Guinea in 1977, each of whom consumed an equivalent of 60-600 ml pure methanol, resulted in all becoming hospitalized within 8-36 h due to acute metabolic acidosis, severe visual impairment and acute pancreatitis. Four died within 72 h after hospitalization. Of 24 who recovered, 16 showed no residual complications, 6 had bilateral visual impairment and 2 had difficulty in speech as well as visual impairment (Dethlefs & Naraqi, 1978; Naraqi et al., 1979).

Before 1978, many alcoholics in Sweden were reported to supplement their intake of alcohol with readily available cleansing solutions containing up to 80% methanol. Since 1978, the methanol content of such solutions has been limited to 5%. However, consumption of these solutions by alcoholics is still widely seen, exposures of 1-2 weeks being associated with blood methanol concentrations ranging from 1000 to 2000 mg/litre (31-62 mmol/litre) (Heath, 1983).

Although ingestion of methanol historically has been shown to be the most frequent route of poisoning, percutaneously absorption of methanol liquids or inhalation of its vapour is as effective as the oral route in producing methanol acute toxic syndrome in adult and pediatric poisonings (Buller & Wood, 1904; Wood & Buller, 1904; Giminez et al., 1968; Kahn & Blum, 1979; Dutkiewicz et al., 1980; Becker, 1983). Giminez et al. (1968) reported 48 children intoxicated with percutaneously applied alcohol. Thirty of these patients had severe respiratory depression, 14 were comatose, 11 had seizures, 7 had anuria or severe oliguria and there were 12 deaths.

About 100 cases of amblyopia (impairment of vision) and death from inhalation of wood alcohol were reported up to 1912, the majority occurring from occupational exposure to the fumes (Tyson & Schoenberg, 1914). Toxicity has also been associated with inhalation of methanol vapour in excess of 400 mg/m^3 (300 ppm) (Becker, 1983; Frederick et al., 1984).

Hazardous inhalation exposures of methanol can occur in the context of intentional inhalation of volatile preparations such as carburettor cleaners. Frenia & Schauben (1993) reported seven cases involving four patients who had inhaled a carburettor cleaner containing toluene (43.8%), methanol (22.3%), methylene chloride (20.5%) and propane (12.5%). Measured blood methanol levels ranged from 504 to 1286 mg/litre. Blood formic acid levels were 120, 193 and 480 μg/ml, respectively, in three patients. Ophthalmic examinations revealed hyperaemic discs and decreased visual acuity in one patient.

Acute methanol toxicity in humans evolves in a fairly defined pattern. A toxic exposure results in a transient mild depression of the CNS, similar to that of ethanol, but to a much lesser degree. The initial depressant period is followed by an asymptotic latent period, which occurs most commonly about 8-24 h after ingestion of the alcohol but may last from several hours to 2 or more days. During the latent period the patients describe no overt symptoms or signs.

The latent period is followed by a syndrome that consists of an uncompensated metabolic acidosis with superimposed toxicity to the visual system. Physical symptoms typically may include headache, dizziness, nausea and vomiting, followed in more severe cases by abdominal and muscular pain and difficult periodic breathing (Kussmaul breathing), which may progress to coma and death, usually from respiratory distress. Death may occur if patients are not treated for metabolic acidosis, and blindness may result even if treatment for metabolic acidosis is performed (Bennett et al., 1953; Röe, 1955; Kane et al., 1968; Tephly & McMartin, 1984; Tephly, 1991).

The neurotoxic effects of methanol on the visual system can involve transient abnormalities such as peripapillary oedema, optic disc hyperaemia, diminished pupillary reactions to light, and central scotomata. Permanent ocular abnormalities include optic disc pallor, attenuation of arterioles, sheathing of arterioles, diminished pupillary reactions to light, diminished visual acuity, central scotomata, and other nerve fibre bundle defects (Bennett et al., 1953; Dethlefs & Naraqi, 1978; Kavet & Nauss, 1990). Pallor of the optic disc is an end-stage sign of irreversible effects of the visual system and may appear 1 to 2 months after an acute methanol dosage (or possibly following chronic occupational exposure to methanol vapour) (Buller & Wood, 1904; Wood & Buller, 1904; Bennett et al., 1953).

Within the general population, the range of the dose levels that is hazardous to humans and the variable susceptibility to acute effects are well recognized (Buller & Wood, 1904; Wood & Buller, 1904; Bennett et al., 1953). As little as 15 ml of 40% methanol resulted in the death of one individual while others survived following the consumption of 500 ml of the same solution in the Atlanta, Georgia, epidemic of 1951. There were large individual differences in the duration of the latency period. Symptoms of methanol poisoning appeared within a few hours or were delayed for up to 72 h. The severity of the disease was not related to the length of the latent period or the amount of methanol consumed (Bennett et al., 1953). (It should be noted that in earlier reported poisoning epidemics, large errors in dose estimates may have been made).

In another example of the range of dose levels of methanol that are toxic, 120 ml (4 fluid ounces) of Columbian spirits, or 95 g of methanol (Columbian spirits is basically pure methanol), was lethal in 40% of the poisoning cases. For a 70-kg person, this dose is equivalent to about 1.4 g methanol/kg body weight (Buller & Wood, 1904). This figure is consistent with currently accepted values for lethality, and 0.3 to 1 g/kg is considered the range of a minimum lethal dose for untreated cases of methanol poisoning (Röe, 1955; Erlanson et al., 1965; Gonda et al., 1978).

It has been suggested that the variability in the reaction to methanol may have been due to the concomitant ingestion of ethanol with methanol, which resulted in some patients having a longer latent period prior to the onset of poisoning (Röe, 1950, 1955). Another explanation for the variability in susceptibility to methanol poisoning is the different levels of folate in the diet. Folate-deficient individuals have a lesser capacity to metabolize formate, so are more susceptible to accumulation of formate to toxic levels (see section 8.1.7 for sensitive sub-populations).

In some clinical cases, the blood methanol level is low in the last phase of the poisoning. In three such cases, blood methanol concentrations were 0.275, 0.277 and 0.194 g/litre, respectively (Erlanson et al., 1965). On the assumption that the body in diffusion equilibrium with the blood represents about 70% of the body weight, Röe (1982) calculated that 0.19-0.14 g/kg of methanol was present in the body. However, low blood methanol levels do not indicate a lower susceptibility to toxicity, i.e., blood methanol levels do not correlate with patient prognosis (Jacobsen & McMartin, 1986). Patients that are examined late after methanol ingestion are likely to have low blood methanol levels, yet high accumulation of formate. Such patients often have poor prognosis.

Acute methanol poisoning patients with blood levels of methanol above 500 mg/litre are generally regarded as requiring haemodialysis (Becker, 1983). The dose of methanol required to achieve this blood concentration is very small (0.4 ml/kg body weight). This corresponds to the ingestion of 4 ml (less than a teaspoon of 100% methanol by a 10-kg (1-year old) child and 28 ml (less than 1 fluid ounce) by a 70-kg adult (Litovitz et al., 1988).

A case was reported of a 46-year-old man who, after consuming a beverage containing methanol, exhibited one of the highest reported serum methanol levels (4930 mg/litre), well above those at which ethanol treatment and haemodialysis are recommended (200 mg/litre and 500 mg/litre, respectively). The lowest serum pH was 7.0 with a hydrogen carbonate level of 8.8 and an anion gap of 42.8. Additionally, his visual acuity decreased to a complete loss of vision. The patient was aggressively treated with haemodialysis and ethanol infusion, regained his vision with a visual acuity of 20/30 bilaterally and suffered no neurological sequelae (Pambies et al., 1993b).

An additional number of cases are particularly informative regarding treatment of methanol intoxication and sequelae of poisoning. A case of methanol intoxication was reported involving a 53-year-old man. Along with blindness and metabolic acidosis, this resulted in cerebral oedema and subarachnoid haemorrhage followed by a comatose state and subsequent death (del Carpio-O'Donavan & Glay, 1992).

A 31-year-old male alcoholic who consumed ethanol containing methanol experienced severe signs and symptoms of poisoning. He underwent minimal medical treatment consisting of sodium hydrogen carbonate and peritoneal dialysis and exhibited necrosis and haemorrhage of the (bilateral) putamen and necrosis of bilateral subcortical white matter and post-contrast gyral enhancement at the otherwise normal-looking areas of the cerebral cortex by the 22nd day, as revealed by computed tomography (Hsieh et al., 1992).

A 31-year-old man entered hospital with a 370 mg/litre serum methanol level after exhibiting the signs and symptoms of methanol poisoning (nausea, vomiting, diffuse abdominal pain and blurred tunnel vision) for 7 days. Following a complete regimen of treatment consisting of hydrogen carbonate, ethanol and folate combined with a 6-h haemodialysis, which corrected the acidosis and eliminated methanol (methanol decreased to 100 mg/litre by the second day), permanent blindness still resulted (Vogt et al., 1993).

A case study of acute methanol poisoning in a 27-year-old man with a previous pattern of drinking was reported by King (1992). Following a comprehensive treatment regimen consisting of administration of alkali, fluids and ethanol, intubation and haemodialysis, this patient exhibited significant neurological and physical impairment, including trauma to the vocal cords and hypophonic voice and urinary incontinence (of central origin), along with cognitive defects. However upon discharge his vision was normal with no atrophy of the optic nerve.

A case of a severe methanol poisoning in a 33-year-old man with a history of alcoholism was reported by Burgess (1992). The individual required 21 h of dialysis to bring the serum methanol levels down to a non-toxic level. A haemodialysis treatment usually lasts approximately 4 h but this may not be sufficient in severe poisoning. Prolonged haemodialysis treatment should be considered in cases of severe poisoning and also possibly for patients with compromised renal function.

Extensive white and grey matter brain damage was seen in an alcoholic 37-year-old man who consumed 1900 ml of windshield washer fluid containing methanol. Both CT scan and MR imaging revealed diffuse white matter oedema and damage throughout frontal and parietal lobes. Bilateral changes in the basal ganglia and necrosis and haemorrhage of putamen were also noted (Glazer & Dross, 1993).

Autopsies from victims of lethal methanol poisonings revealed gross pathology in the visceral organs, the brain, lung, liver, kidney and the CNS, all of which involved a variety of oedematous, haemorrhagic and degenerative changes (Keeney & Mellinkoff, 1951; Bennett et al., 1953; Tonning et al., 1956; Kaplan, 1962; Erlanson et al., 1965; McLean et al., 1980; Wu Chen, 1985; Suit & Estes, 1990).

A fatal case involving a 41-year-old man who had ingested a large quantity of methanol disclosed a broad distribution of methanol in postmortem tissues and fluids. The highest content of methanol was found in the kidney (5.13 g/kg) followed by the liver (4.18 g/kg), vitreous humour (3.9 g/litre), heart (3.45 g/kg), urine (3.43 g/litre), pericardial fluid (3.29 g/litre), blood (2.84 g/litre) and stomach contents (2.21 g/litre) (Pla et al., 1991).

Methanol toxicity can cause brain oedema, necrosis, brain atrophy and cerebral haemorrhage. Putaminal necrosis and haemorrhage result from the direct toxic effects of the methanol metabolites (e.g., formate) and metabolic acidosis in the basal ganglia. The typical appearance of bilateral putaminal necrosis has been described as characteristic of methanol toxicity (Gonda et al., 1978).

Optic neuropathy and putaminal necrosis are the two main complications of methanol poisoning generally occurring in combination after severe poisoning of either suicidal or accidental origin (Sharpe et al., 1982).

A case study of a woman who drank a substantial amount of methylated spirits, which resulted in optic neuropathy and putaminal necrosis, has been reported (Pelletier et al., 1992). The woman exhibited tremor and rigidity, hypokinesia, altered speech and loss of superficial and proprioceptive sensation of the lower extremities with hyperpathia. Signs of moderate bilateral sensory neuropathy and extrapyramidal damage persisted for 2 months as did total blindness due to optic atrophy. Repeat CT and MRI examinations revealed the damage to be a core lesion of the putamen with residual bilateral putaminal hypodensity suggestive of an ischaemic and necrotic process possibly including disruption of the blood-brain barrier.

Postmortem analysis of methanol concentrations in body fluids and tissues reported in fatal human cases of methanol poisoning has revealed higher concentrations of methanol in cerebrospinal fluid (CSF), vitreous humour and bile than in blood (Bennett et al., 1953; Wu Chen et al., 1985). In tissues, the highest concentrations were found in brain, kidney, lung and spleen, and there were lower concentrations in skeletal muscle, pancreas, liver and heart (Wu Chen et al., 1985).

Postmortem signs of damage to the basal ganglia in the brain, specifically the putamen, have been reported in several cases (Erlanson et al., 1965; Aquilonius et al., 1978; Suit & Estes, 1990). A number of human studies have shown that survivors of severe methanol poisoning may suffer residual disorders as a permanent complication (Erlanson et al., 1965; Guggenheim et al., 1971; Aquilonius et al., 1978; McLean et al., 1980; Ley & Gali, 1983). Ley & Gali (1983) described a case of Parkinsonian syndrome after methanol intoxication.

Co-ingestion of methanol with other solvents, e.g., methyl ethyl ketone (MEK) (found in multiple ink cleaning products) has resulted in a hyperosmolar coma without anion gap metabolic acidosis in one reported case of poisoning. MEK was believed to have inhibited methanol metabolism contributing to the low serum formate (1.3 mmol/litre) and normal anion gap despite a blood methanol level of 67 mmol/litre (Price et al., 1994).

8.1.2 Clinical features of acute poisonings

The time course of clinical effects due to acute methanol poisoning is heavily dose-dependent. Blood methanol concentrations of > 500 mg/litre are associated with severe acute clinical signs of toxicity, although formate concentrations may give a better indication of potential toxicity (National Poisons Information Service, 1993).

Thirty minutes to 2 h after ingestion of methanol, clinical effects resemble those of mild ethanol inebriation, and drowsiness, confusion and irritability are often noted. After a latent period, which can range from a few hours to 30 h (but may appear as early as 1 h or as late as 72 h), the patient shows mild CNS depression followed by abdominal pain, nausea, vomiting, hypernoea, gradually failing vision, progressive encephalopathy, severe metabolic acidosis and hypokalaemia; coma and death may ensue. Patients may complain of blurred or "snowfield" vision with whiteness, spots or mistiness within the visual field. Survivors may have permanent blindness or various neurological sequelae. Mortality and morbidity may be more related to the time between ingestion and therapy rather than to the initial methanol levels, thus emphasizing the need for rapid treatment (Mahieu et al., 1989; National Poisons Information Service, 1993; Pambies et al., 1993a).

Metabolic acidosis associated with high anion and osmolal gaps is considered an important laboratory indicator of methanol poisoning (Kruse, 1992). The difference between measured and calculated osmolality or osmolal gap permits a rough estimation of alcohol concentrations (Pappas et al., 1985) so that specific therapy is often initiated before results of quantitative methanol determinations are available.

The determination of osmolal and anion gaps are readily available techniques in the initial handling of poisoning with unknown agents and of patients with a metabolic acidosis of unknown origin. A combined increase in both anion and osmolal gaps has been shown to be a sensitive marker of either ethylene glycol or methanol poisoning (Jacobsen & McMartin, 1986). Reported earlier reference values for osmolal gap and anion gap are -1 (+ 6) mosm/kg H_2O and 16 (+ 2) mmol/litre, respectively (Jacobsen et al., 1982b). However, Aabakken et al. (1994) determined osmolal and anion gaps in populations that were consecutively admitted to a hospital emergency department and suggested that the present reference values for anion and osmolal gaps may be too narrow. They further suggested that the values for the osmolal gap should be 5 + 15 mosm/kg H_2O (-10 to + 20 mosm/kg H_2O) and for the anion gap should be 13 + 9 mmol/litre (4-20 mmol/litre). In their previous reports of methanol poisonings, all patients exceeded these ranges (Jacobsen et al., 1982).

Demedts et al. (1994) hypothesized that excessive serum osmolality gaps that are not predictive of methanol levels as frequently seen in acute poisonings may be attributed to methodology used to measure methanol (analysing samples using head-space GC were compared to results found with gas-chromatography using split-mode injections). Although the determination of increased anion gap is suggestive of methanol poisoning, definitive evidence would be increased blood or serum formate concentrations.

Characteristic clinical and laboratory findings in methanol poisoning are summarized as follows:

* Physical findings
    a) Kussmaul respiration (difficult, periodic breathing)
    b) faint odour of methanol on breath
    c) visual disturbances
    d) nausea, vomiting, abdominal pain
    e) altered sensation

* Laboratory findings
    a) elevated anion gap
    b) metabolic acidosis
    c) elevated osmol gap
    d) positive serum methanol and/or serum formate assay

In treating methanol poisoning a 3-step procedure is common: 1) administration of hydrogen carbonate to combat metabolic acidosis; 2) administration of ethanol to compete as a substrate for alcohol dehydrogenase, and 3) haemodialysis to remove methanol from the blood (Erlanson et al., 1965; Gonda et al., 1978; McCoy et al., 1979; Lins et al., 1980; Jacobsen et al., 1982a,b; Pappas & Silverman, 1982; Becker, 1983; Jacobsen & McMartin, 1986; Kruse, 1992; Pambies et al., 1993a,b). Current recommendations are that ethanol treatment be conducted for patients with blood methanol levels of 200 mg/litre or more, while haemodialysis be used above 500 mg/litre (Jacobsen & McMartin, 1986).

The rationale for the administration of ethanol (Röe, 1950; Keyvan-Larijarni & Tannenbaum, 1974; McCoy et al., 1979; Becker,

1983) is that alcohol dehydrogenase, the enzyme responsible for converting methanol to formaldehyde and formic acid, is also involved in the metabolism of ethanol to acetaldehyde and acetate. The conversion of methanol to its toxic by-products is slowed in the presence of ethanol due to competition for the enzyme.

4-Methyl pyrazole (4-MP) is a more specific inhibitor of alcohol dehydrogenase, less toxic than pyrazole and has been shown to dramatically inhibit production of formic acid from methanol in experimental animals (Blomstrand et al., 1979; McMartin et al., 1980b). Monkeys given usually lethal doses of methanol survived when treated with 4-MP following methanol administration (McMartin et al., 1980b). In humans the slower elimination rate and lesser degree of toxicity of 4-MP suggested that it might be preferable to ethanol in the treatment of methanol poisoning (Jacobsen et al., 1990). 4-MP is currently undergoing clinical trials for treatment of methanol poisoning.

Haemodialysis effectively removes methanol and formate from the circulation (Erlanson et al., 1965; Gonda et al., 1978; McCoy et al., 1979). If haemodialysis is not available, peritoneal dialysis has been used with some success in treating acute methanol intoxication (Keyvan-Larijarnc & Tannenberg, 1974). Discussion of the treatment of methanol poisoning can be found in the IPCS Poisons Information Monograph (PIM) No. 335 (IPCS, 1991).

8.1.3 Repeated or chronic exposure

In comparison to acute toxicity, reports of effects from repeated or chronic methanol exposures have been only infrequently reported. Information based on a limited number of case reports and even fewer epidemiological studies (generally containing unknown levels and/or durations of methanol exposure) suggests that extended exposure to methanol may cause effects qualitatively similar to those observed from relatively high levels of acute exposure, including in some cases CNS and visual disorders (Buller & Wood, 1904; Wood & Buller, 1904; Greenberg et al., 1938; Bennett et al., 1953; Kingsley & Hirsch, 1955; Frederick et al., 1984).

Greenberg et al. (1938) studied 19 workers employed in the production of "fused collars", where solutions of acetone-methanol (3:1) were used to impregnate collars which were then steam-pressed.

Methanol concentrations in the work room were 29-33 mg methanol/m^3 and 96-108 mg acetone/m $.^3$ The shortest period of employment in this occupation was 9 months and the longest was 2 years. No CNS symptoms or visual anomalies were observed.

Frederick et al. (1984) reported on teacher aides who worked at or near spirit duplicators that used a 99% methanol duplicator fluid. The exposures ranged from 1 h/day for 1 day/week to 8 h/day for 5 days/week and had occurred for 3 years. Since the introduction of the equipment, the aides began to experience headaches, dizziness and eye irritation, blurred vision and nausea/upset stomach while working near the machines. Fifteen-minute breathing zone samples near 21 operating machines contained between 475 and 4000 mg/m^3 of methanol vapour. Fifteen of these samples exceeded the NIOSH recommended 15-min standard of 1050 mg/m^3 (800 ppm). The aides were also exposed while collating and stapling papers impregnated with the fluid up to 3 h earlier and these exposures ranged from 235-1140 mg/m^3 . The results suggested that chronic effects may occur when methanol concentrations exceed the threshold limit value (TLV) of 260 mg/m^3 (200 ppm). The effects reported in the study of Frederick et al. (1984) were similar in nature but appeared less severe than those reported from acute poisoning by methanol (Buller & Wood, 1904; Wood & Buller, 1904; Bennett et al., 1953).

Kingsley & Hirsch (1955) reported frequent and persistent headaches, but no visual effects or other permanent sequelae, in clerical workers located close to spirit duplicating equipment that used methanol-based duplicating fluid. Methanol concentrations were reported to be as high as 490 mg/m^3 in the air surrounding the duplicating equipment after 60 min of operation and approximately 130 mg/m^3 about 3 m away from the device. The methanol concentration around the duplicating equipment always exceeded 260 mg/m^3. No information was provided concerning the number of employees exposed or affected, nor on the actual duration of methanol exposure.

NIOSH (1981) reported that 45% of "spirit" duplicating machine operators at the University of Washington experienced some symptoms (blurred vision, headache, nausea, dizziness and eye irritation), consistent with the toxic effects of methanol. Airborne methanol concentrations of 1330 mg/m^3 were measured in the vicinity of the duplicators when windows and doors were open. No information on the actual length of duration of methanol exposure among the employees engaged in the duplicating machine operations were provided.

A number of other studies have measured methanol and formate in the blood and urine of workers exposed during an 8-h day to between 100 and 200 mg/m^3 of methanol vapour (Baumann & Angerer, 1979; Heinrich & Angerer, 1982. Although these studies were predicated on issues of occupational health related to methanol exposure, no health effects were provided nor did the investigators imply that the workers studied had suffered health effects.

Kawai et al. (1991b), utilizing methanol in urine as a biological indicator of occupational exposure, compared subjective complaints and major clinical findings among 33 methanol-exposed workers over several 8-h workshifts. Urine levels of methanol in controls were on average 1.9 ± 0.8 mg/litre (n = 91), and in 14 exposed workers pre-shift concentrations were significantly elevated compared to controls. At the end of the shift the urine concentrations were generally above 100 mg/litre in 8 men with a mean exposure level of 1690 mg/m^3 and 30-100 mg/litre in 6 men with a mean exposure level of 550 mg/m^3. The highest exposures (breathing zone, 8-h/samples) were 4000-7000 mg/m^3 and corresponding urine levels 300-500 mg/litre. The leading subjective complaints included: dimmed vision and nasal irritation during work, and headache, dimmed vision, forgetfulness and increased sensitivity of the skin in the extremities when off-work. The authors attributed the dimmed vision to the fog created by methanol vapours and high humidity in air. No visual problems were noted when windows were kept open and fresh air was allowed to flow in. It was also noted that there were no complaints of photophobia (and thus perhaps no major corneal involvement). Fundus photography revealed that the optic discs were normal and thus the symptom of dimmed vision was not recognized as a sign of impending retinal involvement. In three workers with methanol exposures of 1250-2130 mg/m^3, 1385-2075 mg/m^3 and 155-4685 mg/m^3 (953-1626 ppm, 1058-1585 ppm and 119-3577 ppm) the reaction of pupils to light was slow in two subjects, and a third subject had slight mydriatic pupils. The duration of service of the workers ranged from 0.3 to 7.8 years. The exposures were high and the methods for measurement of visual toxicity were relatively crude, but the data did not indicate that occupational exposure to such concentrations caused permanent damage.

The effects of methanol vapour (249 mg/m^3; SD + 7 mg/m^3) for 75 min on neurobehavioural measures were studied in 12 healthy young men. The exposure produced significant increases (approximately 3 fold) in blood and urine methanol levels but no changes in plasma formate level. Although most of the neurobehavioural end-points were unaffected by exposure to methanol, statistically significant effects and trends were found for a cluster of variables, including the latency of the p-200 component of event-related potentials, performance on the Sternberg memory task and subjective measures of fatigue and concentration. However, the effects were small and did not exceed the normal range (Cook et al., 1991).

.1.4 Reproductive and developmental effects

No studies have been reported in the peer-reviewed literature on the reproductive and developmental effects of methanol in humans.

.1.5 Chromosomal and mutagenic effects

No studies have been reported in the peer-reviewed literature on chromosomal or mutagenic effects of methanol in humans.

.1.6 Carcinogenic effects

No studies have been reported in the literature on the carcinogenicity of methanol in humans.

.1.7 Sensitive sub-populations

Folate-deficient individuals might be at greater risk from inhalation of low concentrations of methanol, compared to normal individuals. Human populations that are potentially at high risk of folate deficiency include pregnant women, the elderly, individuals with poor-quality diets, alcoholics and individuals on certain medications or with certain diseases (API, 1993).

It has been suggested that the metabolic acidosis due to methanol might be exacerbated in individuals with diabetes since it is well known that these patients suffer from diabetic ketoacidosis (Posner, 1975). However, there are no clinical or experimental data on any interaction between methanol acidosis and diabetic ketoacidosis.

9. EFFECTS ON OTHER ORGANISMS IN THE LABORATORY AND FIELD

9.1　Aquatic organisms

9.1.1　Microorganisms

The toxicity of methanol to each of three bacterial groups, i.e., aerobic heterotrophic, Nitrosomonas and methanogens (key agents in the natural recycling of organic material in the environment and in wastewater treatment systems), was described by Blum & Speece (1991). The following IC_{50} values (mg/litre) (the concentration that inhibited the culture by 50%) compared to the uninhibited controls were reported: *Nitrosomonas* (after 24-h exposure), 880 mg/litre; methanogens (after 48-h exposure), 22 000 mg/litre; and aerobic heterotrophs (after 15-h exposure), 20 000 mg/litre. Methanol was found to be completely inhibitory to ammonia oxidation by *Nitrosomonas* bacteria at a concentration of 5×10^{-3} M (about 160 mg/litre) (Hooper & Terry, 1973).

A 15-min EC_{50} of 14 700 mg/litre for the luminescent marine bacterium *Photobacterium phosphoreum* and a 4-h LC_{50} value of 1.0% by volume (7690 mg/litre) have been reported (Schiewe et al., 1985). Calleja et al. (1994) found the EC_{50} for the marine bacterium *Photobacterium phosphoreum* in the Microtox® test to be 29 348 mg/litre. Rajini et al. (1989) reported a 10-min LC_{50} of 6% (44 860 mg/litre) for the ciliate protozoan *Paramecium caudatum*.

Toxicity threshold values for methanol in the cell multiplication inhibition test of 6600 mg/litre for the bacterium *Pseudomonas putida* and > 10 000 mg/litre for the protozoa *Entosiphonsulcatum* were reported by Bringmann & Kühn (1980).

An experimental EC_{50} value (the concentration that reduced the maximum observed biodegradation rate by 50%) for methanol of 2.8 mol/litre (89.7 g/litre) was obtained in a system employing an enriched mixed microbial culture derived from domestic waste water in the USA (Vaishnav & Lopas, 1985).

9.1.2 Algae

Stratton (1987) determined the following EC_{50} values:

Anabaena cylindrica:	2.57% (20 300 mg/litre)
Anabaena inaequalis:	2.68% (21 179 mg/litre)
Anaebaena sp.:	3.12% (24 650 mg/litre)
Anaebaena variabilis:	3.13% (24 730 mg/litre)
Nostoc sp.:	5.48% (43 290 mg/litre)

For the green alga *Chlorella pyrenoidosa* an EC_{50} value of 28 440 mg/litre was found (Stratton & Smith, 1988). Bringman & Kühn (1978), employing a cell multiplication test, reported a toxicity thresholds of 8000 mg/litre for the green alga *Scenedesmus quadricauda* and 530 mg/litre for the cyanobacterium (blue green alga) *Microcystis aeruginosa*.

9.1.3 Aquatic invertebrates

The toxicity of methanol, as reported for a broad spectrum of aquatic invertebrates, is summarized in Table 6. EC_{50} values for the water flea (*Daphnia magna*) range from 13 240 to 24 500 mg/litre. Helmstetter et al. (1996) exposed the mussel, *Mytilus edulis*, to methanol concentrations of 1, 2, 3, 5 and 10% (v/v) for 96 h. All the mussels in both the 5 and 10% exposure groups died within 13.5 h. Sublethal narcotic effects such as slow movement and sporadic filter feeding were reported in mussels exposed to 2 and 3%. Mussels exposed to 1% methanol exhibited no adverse effects during the 96-h exposure period.

9.1.4 Fish

The acute toxicity to fish is listed in Table 7. LC_{50} values reported for freshwater fish species range from 10 880 to 29 700 mg/litre.

The physiological changes in the carp (*Cyprinus carpio*) affected by a sub-lethal methanol concentration of 1 ml/litre (790 mg/litre) included a significant increase in blood cortisol levels after 6 h of exposure, but not after 24 or 72 h, significant decreases in blood protein and cholesterol levels after 72 h of exposure, and reduced concentration of glycogen in the liver after 72 h. Methanol did not produce significant changes in blood glucose levels after any duration of exposure (Gluth & Hanke, 1985).

Table 6. Acute toxicity of methanol to aquatic invertebrates

Organism	Size/age	Stat/flow[a]	Temp (°C)	Hardness (mg/litre)[b]	pH	Parameter[c]	Concentration (mg/litre)[d]		Reference
Water flea (*Daphnia magna*)	<24 h	stat	20	(1)	7.8-8.2	48-h EC_{50}[e]	>10 000	n	Kuhn et al. (1989)
	<24 h	stat	20	(1)	7.8-8.2	48-h EC_0[e]	>10 000	n	Kuhn et al. (1989)
	<24 h	stat	20	(2)	7.8-8.2	24-h EC_{50}	>10 000	n	Bringmann & Kuhn (1982)
	<24 h	stat	20	(2)	7.8-8.2	24-h EC_{100}	>10 000	n	Bringmann & Kuhn (1982)
	<24 h	stat	20	154.5	7.0-8.2	24-h EC_{50}	24 500	n	Bringmann & Kuhn (1982)
						48-h LC_{50}	13 240	n	Vaishnav & Korthals (1990)
						24-h EC_{50}	21 402	n	Calleja et al. (1994)
Water flea (*Daphnia pulex*)	<24 h	stat	22	23±2		18-h-LC_{50}	19 500	n	Bowman et al. (1981)
Water flea (*Daphnia obtusa*)	<24 h	stat	20±2	250	7.8±0.2	24-h EC_{50}	23 500	n	Rossini & Ronco (1996)
	<24 h	stat	20±2	250	7.8±0.2	48-h EC_{50}	22 200	n	

Table 6 (contd).

Species								Reference
Brown shrimp (*Crangon crangon*)	adult	stat	15	seawater	48-h LC_{50}	1975	n	Portmann & Wilson (1971)
	adult	stat*	15	seawater	96-h LC_{50}	1340	n	Portmann & Wilson (1971)
		stat	24.5	seawater	24-h LC_{50}	10 000	n	Price et al. (1974)
Brine shrimp (*Artemia salina*)	24 h	stat	25	seawater	24-h LC_{50}	1578.84	n	Barahona-Gomariz et al. (1994)
	48 h	stat	25	seawater	24-h LC_{50}	1101.46	n	Barahona-Gomariz et al. (1994)
	72 h	stat	25	seawater	24-h LC_{50}	900.73	n	Barahona-Gomariz et al. (1994)
				seawater	24-h LC_{50}	43 574	n	Calleja et al. (1994)
Glass shrimp (*Palaemonetes kadiakensis*)	juvenile	stat	23±2		18 h-LC_{50}	21 900	n	Bowman et al. (1981)
Streptocephalus proboscideus					24-h LC_{50}	32 681	n	Calleja et al. (1994)

Table 6 (contd).

Organism	Size/age	Stat/flow[a]	Temp (°C)	Hardness (mg/litre)[b]	pH	Parameter[c]	Concentration (mg/litre)[d]		Reference
Mussel (*Mytilus edulis*)	5-7 cm	flow	15±0.5	seawater		96-h LC_{50}	15 900	m	Helmstetter et al. (1996)
Cockle (*Cardium edule*)	adult	stat	15	seawater		48-h LC_{50}	7900	n	Portmann & Wilson (1971)
	adult	stat+	15	seawater		96-h LC_{50}	2610-7900	n	Portmann & Wilson (1971)
Harpacticoid, copepod (*Nitocra spinipes*)	adult	stat	21±1	7s	7.9	96-h LC_{50}	12 000	n	Bengtsson et al. (1984)
Scud (*Hyalella azteca*)	juvenile	stat	23±2			18-h LC_{50}	19 350	n	Bowman et al. (1981)
Rotifer (*Brachionus calyciflorus*)						24-h LC_{50}	35 884		Calleja et al. (1994)

[a] stat = static conditions (water unchanged for duration of test); stat* = semi-static conditions (test solutions renewed every 24 h); flow = flow through conditions (concentration of toxicant continuously maintained); s = salinity, expressed as °/₀₀

[b] hardness expressed as mg $CaCO_3$ litre, unless stated otherwise; (1)- total hardness = 2.4 mmol/litre; (2)- total hardness = 2.5 mmol/litre

[c] All EC_{50} values refer to immobilization

[d] n = nominal concentration; m = measured concentration

[e] same as 24 h EC_{50} and EC_0 values

Table 7. Acute toxicity of methanol to fish

Organism	Size/age	Stat/ flow	Temp (°C)	Hardness (mg/litre)[b]	pH	Parameter	Concentration (mg/litre)[c]		Reference
Rainbow trout (*Oncorhynchus mykiss*)	(juv) 0.813 g	flow	12.7±1	46.4	7.0-8.0	24-h EC_{50}[d]	13 200	m	Poirier et al. (1986)
	(juv) 0.813 g	flow	12.7±1	46.4	7.0 - 8.0	96-h EC_{50}[e]	13 000	m	Poirier et al. (1986)
	(juv) 0.813 g	flow	12.7±1	46.4	7.0 - 8.0	24-h LC_{50}	20 300	m	Poirier et al. (1986)
	(juv) 0.813 g	flow	12.7±1	46.4	7.0 - 8.0	96-h LC_{50}[d]	20 100	m	Poirier et al. (1986)
	0.8 g	stat	12	44	7.4	96-h LC_{50}	19 000	n	Mayer & Ellersieck (1986)
	(fingerlings) 1-6 g	flow	12			96-h LC_{50}[d]	20 100	m	US EPA (1983)
Fathead minnow (*Pimephales promelas*)	(28-32 d) 0.126 g	flow	23.3±1.7	46.4	7.0-8.0	24-h EC_{50}[d]	29 700	m	Poirier et al. (1986)
	(28-32 d) 0.126 g	flow	23.3±1.7	46.4	7.0-8.0	96-h EC_{50}[e]	28 900	m	Poirier et al. (1986)
	(28-32 d) 0.126 g	flow	23.3±1.7	46.4	7.0-8.0	24-h LC_{50}[d]	29 700	m	Poirier et al. (1986)

Table 7 (contd).

Organism	Size/age	Stat/ flow	Temp (°C)	Hardness (mg/litre)[b]	pH	Parameter	Concentration (mg/litre)[c]		Reference
Fathead minnow (*Pimephales promelas*)	(28-32 d) 0.126 g	flow	23.3±1.7	46.4	7.0-8.0	96-h LC_{50}	29 400	m	Poirier et al. (1986)
	(30 d) 0.12 g	flow	24-26	45.5	7.5	96-h LC_{50}	28 100	m	Veith et al. (1983)
Bluegill sunfish (*Leponimis macrochirus*)	(juv) 3.07 g	flow	19.8±2.3	46.4	7.0-8.0	24-h EC_{50}[e]	16 100	m	Poirier et al. (1986)
	(juv) 3.07 g	flow	19.8±2.3	46.4	7.0-8.0	24-h EC_{50}[e]	16 100	m	Poirier et al. (1986)
	(juv) 3.07 g	flow	19.8±2.3	46.4	7.0-8.0	48-h EC_{50}[e]	16 000	m	Poirier et al. (1986)
	(juv) 3.07 g	flow	19.8±2.3	46.4	7.0-8.0	96-h EC_{50}[e]	12 700	m	Poirier et al. (1986)
	(juv) 3.07 g	flow	19.8±2.3	46.4	7.0-8.0	24-h LC_{50}[d]	19 100	m	Poirier et al. (1986)
	(juv) 3.07 g	flow	19.8±2.3	46.4	7.0-8.0	96-h LC_{50}	15 400	m	Poirier et al. (1986)
	1.5 g	flow	25			24-h LC_{50}[d]	19 230	m	US EPA (1983)
	1.5 g	flow	25			96-h LC_{50}	15 500	m	US EPA (1983)

Table 7 (contd).

Species	Age/size	Test	Temp (°C)	Hardness	pH	Endpoint	Value		Reference
Guppy (*Poecilia reticulata*)	2-3 months	stat[*]	21-23	25		7-day LC_{50}	10 860	m	Konemann (1981)[g] Hermens & Leeuwangh (1982)
Golden orfe (*Leuciscus idus melanotus*)	juv	stat	19-21	(1)	7.0 -8.0	48-h LC_{50}	>10 000[f]	m	Juhnke & Lüdemann (1978)
	juv	stat	19-21	(1)	7.0 -8.0	48-h LC_0	7900[f]	m	Juhnke & Lüdemann (1978)
	juv	stat	19-21	(1)	7.0 -8.0	48-h LC_{100}	>10 000[f]	m	Juhnke & Lüdemann (1978)

Table 7 (contd).

Organism	Size/age	Stat/flow	Temp (°C)	Hardness (mg/litre)[b]	pH	Parameter	Concentration (mg/litre)[c]	Reference
Bleak (*Alburnus alburnus*)	8 cm	stat	10	7s	7.9	96-h LC_{50}	28 000 n	Bengtsson et al. (1984)
Armed bullhead (*Agonus cataphractus*)	adult	stat*	15	seawater		96-h LC_{50}[d]	7900-26 070 n	Portmann & Wilson (1971)

[a] stat = static conditions (water unchanged for duration of test)
stat* = semi-static conditions (test solutions renewed every 24 hours)
flow = flow through conditions (concentration of toxicant continuously maintained)
s = salinity, expressed as $^{0}/_{00}$
[b] hardness expressed as $mg/CaCO_3/litre$, unless otherwise stated; (1)- total hardness = 2.7 mmol/litre;
[c] n = nominal concentration
m = measured concentration
[d] same as 48-h LC_{50} or EC_{50} values
[e] effects on equilibrium, behaviour and coloration
[f] two laboratories following the same test protocol, same result from each laboratory
[g] consulted for experimental method only

The effect of methanol on the fertilization of chum salmon (*Oncorhynchus keta*) ova was examined at methanol exposure levels of 0.001% to 10% by volume (7.9 to 79 000 mg/litre) (Craig et al., 1977). Both gametes (sperm and unfertilized ova) and fertilized eggs were exposed to methanol for brief periods. Exposures up to and including 1% methanol did not significantly affect fertilization, survival to hatching, hatching time, alevin size at hatch or physical deformities among alevins, although a methanol concentration of 10% was lethal in most cases (Craig et al., 1977).

Cuéllar et al. (1995) determined the effect of methanol on the embryonic development of the medaka fish (*Oryzias latipes*). The eggs were exposed to methanol in both Petri dishes and vials. No effects on embryonic development were reported at a methanol concentration of 0.5%.

9.2 Terrestrial organisms

9.2.1 *Plants*

Hemming et al. (1995) determined the effect of methanol on the respiration of pepper (*Capsicum annuum*), tomato (*Lycopersicon esulentum*) and petunia (*Petunia hybrida*). Whole plants were exposed to either methanol vapour or methanol solution. The general response to methanol was the same for the three species, with a respiratory rate increase of up to 50% at the lower methanol concentrations tested. The response was the same for exposure to methanol vapour or solution. Exposure of a single leaf resulted in a systemic response throughout the whole plant within a few hours. The response lasted for several weeks. Decreased metabolic rates and waterlogged appearance were reported in plants following a brief exposure of a leaf to methanol concentrations ≥ 30%. Root tissue was reported to be more sensitive; a decrease in metabolic rate was reported following brief exposures to ≥ 10% methanol.

10. EVALUATION OF EFFECTS ON HUMAN HEALTH AND THE ENVIRONMENT

10.1 Evaluation of human health risks

10.1.1 Exposure

Methanol occurs naturally in humans, animals and plants. Humans are routinely exposed to low levels of methanol from both the diet (fruits, vegetables, fruit juices and foods containing the synthetic sweetener aspartame) and metabolic processes. Human exposure to large acutely toxic amounts of methanol via the oral route has principally been noted in a relatively small number of individuals, generally resulting through accidental or intentional consumption of methanol in illicit or contaminated alcoholic beverages.

Methanol is produced in large amounts in many countries and is extensively used as an industrial solvent, a chemical intermediate (principally in the production of methyl tertiary butyl ether (MTBE), formaldehyde, acetic acid and glycol ethers), as a denaturant of ethanol and in a variety of consumer products.

The most important route of occupational exposure to methanol is inhalation. Sources of occupational exposure include the dissipative emissions of methanol primarily occurring from miscellaneous solvent usage, methanol production, end-product manufacturing and bulk storage and handling.

An increased number of people could be potentially exposed to environmental methanol as a result of the projected expanded use of methanol in methanol-blended gasolines. Exposures would principally arise from exhaust, evaporative emissions and normal heating of the engine. Simulation models based on 100% of all vehicles powered by methanol-based fuels predict concentrations of methanol in urban streets, expressways, railroad tunnels or parking garages ranging from a low of 1 mg/m^3 (0.77 ppm) to a high of 60 mg/m^3 (46 ppm). Predicted concentrations during refuelling of vehicles range from 30 to 50 mg/m^3 (23-38.5 ppm). For comparison and reference purposes, a current occupational exposure limit for methanol in many countries is 260 mg/m^3 (200 ppm) for an 8-h working day.

There are limited data on human dermal exposure to methanol but the potential expanded use of methanol in automotive fuels would increase the potential for dermal exposure in a large number of people.

10.1.2 Human health effects

Methanol is rapidly absorbed by inhalation, ingestion and dermal exposure and is rapidly distributed to tissues according to the distribution of body water. The dose and blood concentrations of methanol and its metabolite formate are among the major determinants of the resultant toxicity in humans.

The acute and short-term toxicity of methanol varies greatly between different species, toxicity being highest in species with a relatively poor ability to metabolize formate. Methanol has been studied most intensively in acute high-dose oral exposures in laboratory animals and as case reports of ingestion in humans. In general, humans and primates respond to such exposures with transient central nervous system (CNS) depression (intoxication), followed by an asymptomatic latent period culminating in metabolic acidosis and severe ocular toxicity (blindness).

Non-primate animals such as rodents do not ordinarily exhibit metabolic acidosis or blindness on exposure to methanol although they exhibit the general narcotic effects noted in non-human primates and humans. The clearance of formate from the blood of exposed primates is at least 50% slower than in rodents. Formate, an endogenous biological substrate, is detoxified by a multi-step pathway to CO_2 via a tetrahydrofolate (THF)-dependent pathway. Species such as rodents with high hepatic THF levels are less sensitive to the toxic effects of methanol than species with low hepatic THF levels such as humans and non-human primates. The faster rate of formate removal means that rodents do not accumulate formate above endogenous levels and hence are not susceptible to methanol-induced metabolic acidosis or ocular toxicity.

The primary enzymatic pathway that catalyses methanol metabolism in humans and non-human primates is alcohol dehydrogenase, while in the rat it is the catalase-peroxidase system. Available data suggest that methanol elimination from the systemic circulation is capacity-limited in both rats and in humans.

Studies in humans and non-human primates exposed to concentrations of methanol ranging from 13 to 2601 mg/m³ (10 to 2001 ppm) and the widely used occupational exposure limit of 260 mg/mg³ (200 ppm) suggest that exposure to methanol vapour during the normal use of methanol fuel does not pose an unacceptable risk to healthy adults. General population exposures to methanol through air (although infrequently measured) are over 1000 times lower than occupational limits.

Along with methanol, formate is present in blood at low endogenous concentrations, being found naturally in some foods and also produced as a by-product of several metabolic pathways, including histidine and tryptophan degradation. Background levels of formate in humans have been shown to range from 3 to 19 mg/litre (0.07-0.4 mM).

Human susceptibility to the acute effects of methanol intoxication are extremely variable. On the basis of available human case reports, the minimum lethal dose in the absence of medical treatment is in the range of 0.3 to 1 g/kg. The major determinants of human susceptibility to methanol toxicity appear to be the concurrent ingestion of ethanol, which slows the entrance of methanol into the metabolic pathway, and the hepatic status of THF, which governs the rate of formate detoxification.

Some human populations are at increased risk of folate deficiency. These include pregnant women, the elderly, individuals with poor-quality diets, alcoholics, and individuals on certain medications or with certain diseases.

Much fewer data are available on the health effects in humans or laboratory animals associated with chronic or repeated exposure to methanol. In the absence of details of exposure (e.g., duration, concentrations), the effects of prolonged exposure are considered qualitatively very similar to those reported for acute cases, ranging from nausea and dizziness to blurred vision and temporary or permanent blindness. Chronic exposure to methanol vapour concentrations of 480-4000 mg/m³ (365-3080 ppm) has resulted in headache, dizziness, nausea and blurred vision.

There are no reports of carcinogenic, genotoxic, reproductive or developmental effects in humans due to methanol exposures.

10.1.3 Approaches to assessment of risk

The assessment of risk from chronic exposure requires dose-response information in the form of quantitative data from animal studies using appropriate test species and, where available, relevant human epidemiological and clinical data. In the case of methanol, the assessment of the risks of exposure is confounded by the fact that both methanol and its toxic metabolite, formate, are endogenous metabolic intermediates in all species including humans. Therefore, it must be assumed that there are levels of methanol exposure that do not represent significant risk. Determining the hazards associated with methanol exposure is additionally complicated by the fact that there are no adequate or comprehensive data from animal tests for chronic toxicity. Because of species differences in methanol metabolism, data available from normal rats appear to be inappropriate for use in characterizing the adverse effects of methanol in humans. Investigation of folate-deficient rodent models may provide valuable mechanistic, pharmacokinetic and toxicological effect information on methanol, particularly with respect to acute exposures. However, the nature of this animal model is such that it may have inherent weaknesses for the toxicological assessment of long-term exposure because of the adverse effects of folate deficiency itself and the background nutritional status of these rats in chronic studies. Similarities in the metabolism of methanol within primates suggest the use of non-human primates may be more appropriate for determining the nature of the hazards of methanol for humans, but adequate findings for chronic exposure are also lacking. Human methanol exposure data are extensive but primarily focus on acute exposure and clinical effects associated with poisoning. Although this information from humans does highlight the wide individual variability in the toxic response to methanol in humans, it contains limited comprehensive information on sub-chronic to chronic methanol exposure.

Taken together, the above considerations suggest a conventional safety or risk assessment would not appear feasible, and would most likely be incomplete at present. An alternative approach might be one based on consideration of blood levels of the most toxic metabolite, formate. Since formate occurs naturally in humans, it would seem reasonable to assume that normal background levels should not pose any risk to health and consequently that levels of human exposure that do not result in levels of blood formate above background levels could be considered to pose insignificant risk. In this respect, based on information from limited studies in humans, it might be concluded that occupational exposure to current exposure limits (around 260 mg/m^3) or single oral exposure to approximately 20 mg/kg body weight would fall into this category.

10.2 Evaluation of effects on the environment

Methanol may be released into the environment in significant amounts during its production, storage, transportation and use.

Methanol is readily degraded in the environment by photo-oxidation. Half-lives of 7-18 days have been reported for the atmospheric reaction of methanol with hydroxyl radicals.

Methanol is readily biodegradable under both aerobic and anaerobic conditions in a wide variety of environmental media. Many genera and strains of microorganisms are capable of using methanol as a growth substrate. Generally 80% of methanol in sewage systems is biodegraded within 5 days.

Methanol is a normal growth substrate for many soil microorganisms, which are capable of completely degrading methanol to carbon dioxide and water.

Methanol is of low toxicity to aquatic and terrestrial organisms and it is not bioaccumulated. Effects due to environmental exposure to methanol are unlikely to be observed, unless it is released to the environment in large quantities, such as a spill.

In summary, unless released in high concentrations, methanol would not be expected to persist or bioaccumulate in the environment. Low levels of release would not be expected to result in adverse environmental effects.

11. RECOMMENDATIONS FOR PROTECTION OF HUMAN HEALTH AND THE ENVIRONMENT

11.1 Protection of human health

a) Methanol and methanol mixtures should be clearly labelled with a warning of the acute toxicity of methanol. Labels should use the description "methanol".

b) Storage, process and drying plants should be designed to protect against fire and explosion risks and exposure of personnel to methanol.

c) Workplaces where methanol is present should be provided with adequate ventilation to minimize inhalation exposure. Where necessary, personnel handling methanol should be provided with suitable protective clothing to prevent skin contamination.

d) Clinicians should be aware of the latent period and signs and symptoms following exposure to methanol, particularly by ingestion. Consideration associated with the existence of sensitive subgroups should be recognized, including those at increased risk of folate deficiency.

e) To avoid misuse, methanol used as fuel should be denatured and should contain a colour additive.

11.2 Protection of the environment

Although methanol is rapidly degraded in the environment and is of low acute toxicity to aquatic organisms, care should be taken to prevent spills of large quantities of methanol. Particular care should be taken to prevent spilled methanol reaching surface water.

12. FURTHER RESEARCH

a)   Further research is needed to characterize the mechanism and pathogenesis of methanol-induced visual toxicity.

b)   There is a need for definitive studies concerning the dose-response relationship for subtle CNS function using neurotoxic, neurobehavioural and ocular end-points across species at both single and repeated low-level exposures.

c)   Investigation of the metabolism of methanol and formate in target organs, including the brain, retina, optic nerve and testes, under various exposure conditions is needed.

d)   The pharmacokinetics of methanol and formate during pregnancy should be investigated in appropriate animal models to determine whether long-term exposure to methanol alters maternal or fetal disposition of methanol and formate.

e)   Additional studies are required to resolve whether methanol, formate or a combination of the two is responsible for methanol-induced developmental toxicity.

f)   Exposure models should be developed and validated to estimate exposure concentrations and routes of exposure in specific exposure scenarios. Ambient and personal monitoring to determine the distribution of exposures should be conducted.

g)   Dose-effect and time-course relationships for both acute and chronic effects of methanol or formate generated from methanol, in humans or appropriate models, have not been established and are essential for adequate risk assessment.

h)   There is a need for studies into the nutritional, metabolic, genetic and age-related factors that may contribute to variation in susceptibility to methanol intoxication.

i)   The genotoxic effects of methanol should be further investigated to determine whether it is clastogenic.

j) A rapid, practical and inexpensive assay for formate in blood and body tissues is needed for early diagnosis of methanol poisoning.

k) Improved therapeutic measures, including the development of 4-methylpyrazole and new agents for reversing formate-induced visual neurotoxicity, are needed.

13. PREVIOUS EVALUATION BY INTERNATIONAL BODIES

Methanol was evaluated in 1970 as an extraction solvent by the Joint FAO/WHO Expert Committee on Food Additives.

The Committee recommended that when used as an extraction solvent, residues should be reduced to a minimum by observing good manufacturing practice. It was considered that the limited uses of methanol as an extraction solvent for spice and hop oils meant that residues from these sources were insignificant in the diet (FAO/WHO, 1971; WHO, 1971).

REFERENCES

Aabakken L, Johansen KS, Rydningen EB, Bredesen JE, Ovrebos S, & Jacobsen D (1994) Osmolal and anion gaps in patients admitted to an emergency medical department. Hum Exp Toxicol, **13**: 131-134.

Abbondandolo A, Bonatti S, Corsi C, Corti G, Fiorio R, Leporini C, Mazzacccaro A, & Nieri R (1980) The use of organic solvents in mutagenicity testing. Mutat Res, **79**: 141-150.

Abbott BD, Logsdon TR, & Wilke TS (1994) Effects of methanol on embryonic mouse palate in serum-free organ culture. Teratology, **49**: 122-134.

Abbott BD, Ebron-McCoy M, & Andrews JE (1995) Cell death in rat and mouse embryos exposed to methanol in whole embryo culture. Toxicology, **97**: 159-171.

Agarwal VK (1988) Determination of low relative molecular mass alcohols in gasoline by gas chromatography. Analyst, **113**: 907-909.

Akimoto H & Takagi H (1986) Formation of methyl nitrite in the surface reaction of nitrogen dioxide and methanol: 2. Photoenhancement. Environ Sci Technol, **20**: 393-397.

Allis JW, Simmons JE, Robinson BL, McDonald A, & House DE (1992) Induction of rat hepatic cytochrome P-450II E1 by methanol: Its role in the enhancement of carbon tetrachloride hepatotoxicity. Toxicologist, **12**: 85.

Allis JW, Brown BL, Simmons JE, Hatch GE, McDonald A, & House DE (1996) Methanol potentiation of carbon tetrachloride hepato toxicity: the central role of cytochrome P450. Toxicology, **112**: 131-170.

Anderson EV (1993) Health studies indicate MTBE is safe gas additive. Chem Eng News, **71**(38): 9-18.

Andrews LS, Clary JJ, Terrill JB, & Bolte HF (1987) Subchronic inhalation toxicity of methanol. J Toxicol Environ Health, **20**: 117-124.

Andrews JE, Ebron-McCoy M, Logsdon TR, Mole LM, Kavlock RJ, & Rogers JM (1993) Developmental toxicity of methanol in whole embryo culture: A comparative study with mouse and rat embryos. Toxicology, **81**: 205-215.

Andrews JE, Ebron-McCoy M, Kavlock RJ, & Rogers JM (1995) Developmental toxicity of formate and formic acid in whole embryo culture: A comparative study with mouse and rat embryos. Teratology, **51**: 243-251.

Angerer J & Lehnert G (1977) Occupational exposure to methanol. Acta Pharmacol, **41**: 551-556.

Anon (1991) Methanol: tight markets ahead. Chem Ind, **17**: 598.

AOAC (1980) In: Horwitz W ed. Official methods of analysis of the Association of Official Analytical Chemists, 13th ed. Washington, DC, Association of Official Analytical Chemists, pp 9.107, 9.086-9.093.

AOAC (1990) In: Helrich K ed. Official methods of analysis of the Association of Official Analytical Chemists, 15th ed. Washington, DC, Association of Official Analytical Chemists, pp 702-705.

API (1993) Study of the relationship between folate studies and methanol toxicity. Washington, DC, American Petroleum Industry (Publication No. 4554).

Aquilonius S, Askmark H, Enoksson P, Lundberg PO, & Mostrom U (1978) Computerized tomography in severe methanol intoxication. Br Med J, **ii**: 929-930.

ASTM (1993) Standard test methods for the determination of MTBE, ETBE, TAME, DIPE, tert-amyl alcohol and C_1 to C_4 alcohols in gasoline by gas chromatography (D4815). Philadelphia, Pennsylvania, American Society for Testing and Materials.

ATSDR (Agency for Toxic Substances Disease Registry) (1993) Methanol toxicity. Am Fam Phys, **47**: 163-174.

Auto/Oil Air Quality Improvement Research Program (1992) Emissions and air quality modeling results from methanol/gasoline blends and prototype flexible/variable vehicles. Atlanta, Georgia, US Gasoline Producers, Coordinating Research Council (Technical Bulletin No.7).

Auto/Oil Air Quality Improvement Research Program (1994) Emissions from methanol fuels and reformulated gasoline in 1993 production flexible/variable fuel and gasoline vehicles (Technical Bulletin No. 13).

Axelrod J & Daly J (1965) Pituitary gland : enzymic formation of methanol from S-adenosylmethionine. Science, **158**: 892-993.

Baker RN, Alenty Al, & Zack JF Jr (1969) Simultaneous determination of lower alcohols, acetone and acetaldeyhde in blood by gas chromatography. J Chromatogr Sci, **7**: 312-314.

Barahona-Gomariz MV, Sanz-Barrera F, & Sánchez-Fortún S (1994) Acute toxicity of organic solvents on *Artemia salina*. Bull Environ Contam Toxicol, **52**: 766-771.

Barnes I, Bastian V, Becker KH, Fink EH, & Zabel F (1982) Reactivity studies of organic substances towards hydroxyl radicals under atmospheric conditions. Atmos Environ, **16**: 545-550.

Bartlett GR (1950) Inhibition of methanol oxidation by ethanol in the rat. Am J Physiol, **163**: 619-621.

BASF (1979) [Report on the comparative testing on sensitizing effects in guinea pigs, modified maximization test.] Ludwigshafen, Germany, BASF AG, 11 pp (Unpublished report) (in German).

BASF (1980a) [Determination of the acute inhalation toxicity LD_{50} of methanol (Merck min. 99.8%) as vapour at 4 hours exposure to Sprague-Dawley rats.] Ludwigshafen, Germany, BASF AG, 14 pp (Unpublished report) (in German).

BASF (1980b) [Determination of the acute inhalation toxicity LD_{50} of methanol (Merck min. 99.8%) as vapour at 6 hours exposure to Sprague-Dawley rats.] Ludwigshafen, Germany, BASF AG, 22 pp (Unpublished report) (in German).

Baumann K & Angerer J (1979) Occupational chronic exposure to organic solvents: VI. Formic acid concentration in blood and urine as an indicator of methanol exposure. Int Arch Occup Environ Health, **42**: 241-249.

Baumbach GI, Cancilla PA, Martin-Amat G, Tephly TR, McMartin KE, Makar Ab, Hayreh M, & Haryeh SS (1977) Methyl alcohol poisoning: IV. Alterations of the morphological findings of the retina and optic nerve. Arch Ophthalmol, **95**: 1859-1865.

Becker CE (1983) Methanol poisoning. J Emerg Med, **1**: 51-58.

Bellar TA & Sigsby JE Jr (1970) Direct gas chromatographic analysis of low molecular weight substituted organic compounds in emissions. Environ Sci Technol, **4**: 150-156.

Bengtsson BE, Renberg L, & Tarkpea M (1984) Molecular structure and aquatic toxicity-an example with C_1-C_{13} aliphatic alcohols. Chemosphere, **13**(5/6): 613-622.

Bennett IL, Cary FH, Mitchell GL, & Cooper MN (1953) Acute methyl alcohol poisoning: a review based on experiences in an outbreak of 323 cases. Medicine, **32**: 431-463.

Benoit FM, Davidson WR, Lovett AM, Nacson S, & Ngo A (1985) Breath analysis by API/MS-human exposure to volatile organic solvents. Int Arch Occup Environ Health, **55**: 113-120.

Bindler F, Voges E, & Laugel P (1988) The problem of methanol concentration admissible in distilled fruit spirits. Food Addit Contam, **5**: 343-351.

Blanch GP, Tabera J, Sanz J, Herraiz M, & Reglero G (1992) Volatile composition of vinegars. Simultaneous distillation-extraction and gas chromatographic-mass spectrometric analysis. J Agric Chem, **40**: 1046-1049.

Blomstrand R, Ostling-Wintzell H, Lof A, McMartin K, Tolf BR, & Hedstrom KG (1979) Pyrazoles as inhibitors of alcohol oxidation and as important tools in alcohol research: an approach to therapy against methanol poisoning. Proc Natl Acad Sci (USA), **76**: 3499-3503.

Blum DJW & Speece RE (1991) A data base of chemical toxicity to environmental bacteria and its use in interspecies comparisons and correlations. Res J Water Pollut Control Fed, **63**: 198-207.

Bock JL (1982) Analysis of serum by high-field proton nuclear magnetic resonance. Clin Chem, **28**: 1873-1877.

Boeniger MF (1987) Formate in urine as a biological indicator of formaldehyde exposure: a review. Am Ind Hyg Assoc J, **48**: 900-908.

Bolon B, Dorman DC, Janszen D, Morgan KT, & Welsch F (1993) Phase specific developmental toxicity in mice following maternal methanol inhalation. Fundam Appl Toxicol, **21**: 508-516.

Bolon B, Welsch F, & Morgan KT (1994) Methanol induced neural tube defects in mice: pathogenesis during neuralation. Teratology, **49**: 497-517.

Boos RN (1948) Quantitative colorimetric microdetermination of methanol with chromotropic acid. Anal Chem, **20**: 964-965.

Bowman MC, Oller WL, Cairns T, Gosnell AB, & Oliver KH (1981) Stressed bioassay systems for rapid screening of pesticide residues. Part I: Evaluation of bioassay systems. Arch Environ Contam Toxicol, **10**: 9-24.

Braun M & Stolp H (1985) Degradation of methanol by a sulfate reducing bacterium. Arch Microbiol, **142**: 77-80.

Bresnick GH (1989) Excitotoxins: A possible new mechanism for the pathogenesis of ischemic retinal damage. Arch Ophthalmol, **107**: 339-341.

Bringmann G & Kühn R (1980) Comparison of the toxicity thresholds of water pollutants to bacteria, algae and protozoa in the cell multiplication inhibition test. Water Res, **14**: 231-241.

Buller F & Wood CA (1904) Poisoning by wood alcohol. J Am Med Assoc, **43**: 1058-1062.

Burbacher TM (1993) Neurotoxic effects of gasoline and gasoline constituents. Environ Health Perspect, **101**(Suppl 6): 133-141.

Burgess E (1992) Prolonged hemodialysis in methanol intoxication. Pharmacotherapy, **12**: 238-239.

Buttery JE & Chamberlain BR (1988) A simple enzymatic method for the measurement of abnormal levels of formate in plasma. J Anal Toxicol, **12**: 292-294.

Calleja MC, Persoone G, & Geladi P (1994) Comparative acute toxicity of the first 50 multicentre evaluation of *in vitro* cytotoxicity chemicals to aquatic non-vertebrates. Arch Environ Contam Toxicol, **26**: 69-78.

Cameron AM, Nilsen OG, Haug E, & Eik-Nes KB (1984) Circulating concentrations of testosterone, luteinizing hormone and follicle stimulating hormone in male rats after inhalation of methanol. Arch Toxicol, **7**(Suppl): 441-443.

Cameron AM, Zahlsen K, Haug E, Nilsen OG, & Eik-Nes KB (1985) Circulating steroids in male rats following inhalation of n-alcohols. Arch Toxicol, **8**(Suppl): 422-424.

Campbell JA, Howard DR, Backer LC, & Allen JW (1991) Evidence that methanol inhalation does not induce chromosome damage in mice. Mutat Res, **260**: 257-264.

Casey JC, Self R, & Swain T (1963) Origin of methanol and dimethyl sulfide from cooked foods. Nature (Lond), **200**: 885.

Cavanaugh LA, Schadt CF, & Robinson E (1969) Atmospheric hydrocarbon and carbon monoxide measurements at Point Barrow, Alaska. Environ Sci Technol, **3**: 251-257.

CEC (Commission of the European Communities) (1988) Solvents in common use: Health risks to workers. Cambridge, Royal Society of Chemistry, pp 1-7, 157-186 (Publication EUR/11553).

Chang TY & Rudy SJ (1990) Ozone-forming potential of organic emissions from alternative-fueled vehicles. Atmos Environ, **24A**: 2421-2430.

Chang LW, McMillan L, Wynne BR, Pereira MA, Colley RA, Ward JB, & Legator MS (1983) The evaluation of six monitors from the exposure to formaldehyde in laboratory animals. Environ Mutagen, **5**: 381-387.

Chao CT (1959) [Data for determining the standard maximum permissible concentration of methanol vapours in the atmospheric air.] Gig I Sanit, **24**: 7-12 (in Russian).

Cheung ST & Lin WN (1987) Simultaneous determination of methanol, ethanol, isopropanol and ethylene glycol in plasma by gas chromatography. J Chromatogr, **414**: 248-250.

Clark CB, Dutcher JS, McClellan RG, Naman TM, & Seizinger DE (1983) Influence of ethanol and methanol gasoline blends on the mutagenicity of particulate exhaust extracts. Arch Environ Contam Toxicol, **12**: 311-317.

Clay KL, Murphy RC, & Watkins WD (1975) Experimental methanol toxicity in the primate: analysis of metabolic acidosis. Toxicol Appl Pharmacol, **34**: 49-61.

Clayton GD & Clayton FE ed. (1982) Patty's industrial hygiene and toxicology - Volume 2C: Toxicology with cumulative index for Volume 2, 3rd ed. New York, Chichester, Brisbane, Toronto, John Wiley & Sons, pp 4527-4551.

Coe JI & Sherman RE (1970) Comparative study of postmortem vitreous ..... and blood alcohol. J Forensic Sci, **25**: 185-190.

Coleman EC, Ho CT, & Chang SS (1981) Isolation and identification of volatile compounds from baked potatoes. J Agric Food Chem, **29**: 42-48.

CONCAWE (1995) Alternative fuels in the automotive market. Brussels, CONCAWE, 67 pp (Report No. 2/95, prepared for the CONCAWE Automotive Emissions Management Group by its Technical Coordinator, RC Hutcheson).

Cook WA (1945) Maximum allowable concentrations of industrial atmospheric contaminants. Ind Med, **14**: 936-946.

Cook MR, Bergman FJ, Cohen HD, Gerkovich MM, Graham O, Harris RX, & Siemann LG (1991) Effects of methanol vapor on human neurobehavioural measures. Cambridge, Massachusetts, Health Effects Institute (Research Report No. 42).

Cooper JR & Felig P (1961) The biochemistry of methanol poisoning: II. Metabolic acidosis in the monkey. Toxicol Appl Pharmacol, **3**: 202-209.

Cooper RL, Rehnberg GL, Goldman JM, Linder RE, Mole ML, Edwards TL, Hein JF, & McElroy WK (1990) Effect of methanol on hormonal control of testes in male rats. Toxicologist, **10**: 211.

Cooper RI, Mole ML, Rehnberg GL, Goldman JM, McElroy WK, Hein J, & Stoker TE (1992) Effects of inhaled methanol on pituitary and testicular hormones in chamber acclimated and non-acclimated rats. Toxicology, **71**: 69-81.

Costantini MG (1993) Health effects of oxygenated fuels. Environ Health Perspect, **101**(Suppl 6): 151-160.

Craig PC, Withler FC, & Morley RB (1977) Effects of methanol on the fertilization of chum salmon (*Oncorhynchus keta*) ova. Environ Pollut, **14**: 85-91.

Crebelli R, Conti G, Conti L, & Carere A (1989) A comparative study on ethanol and acetaldehyde as inducers of chromosome malsegregation in *Aspergillus nidulans*. Mutat Res, **215**: 187-195.

Creel DJ, Dustman RD, & Beck EC (1970) Differences in visually evoked responses in albino versus hooded rats. Exp Neurol, **29**: 298-309.

Cuéllar M, González M, & Muñoz MJ (1995) [Methanol toxicity on the embryonic development of *Oryzias latipes*.] Rev Toxicol, **12**: 109-113 (in Spanish).

Cummings AM (1993) Evaluation of the effects of methanol during early pregnancy in the rat. Toxicology, **79**: 205-214.

D'Alessandro A, Osterloh JD, Chuwers P, Quinlan PJ, Kelly TJ, & Becker CE (1994) Formate in serum and urine after controlled methanol exposure at the threshold limit value. Environ Health Perspect, **102**: 178-181.

Damian P & Rabbe OG (1996) Toxicokinetic modelling of dose-dependent formate elimination in rats: *in vivo-in vitro* correlations using perfused rat liver. Toxicol Appl Pharmacol, **139**: 22-32.

Davoli E, Cappellini L, Airoldi L, & Fanelli R (1986) Serum methanol concentrations in rats and in men after a single dose of aspartame. Food Chem Toxicol, **24**: 187-189.

De Flora S, Zanacchi P, Camoirano A, Bennicelli C, & Badolati GS (1984) Genotoxic activity and potency of 135 compounds in the Ames reversion test and in a bacterial DNA-repair test. Mutat Res, **133**: 161-198.

Deichmann WB (1948) Methanol. J Ind Hyg Toxicol, **30**: 373-376.

Del Carpio-O'Donovan L & Glay J (1992) Subarachnoid hemorrhage resulting from methanol intoxication: Demonstrated by computed tomography. Can Assoc Radiol J, **43**: 263-299.

Demedts P, Theunis L, Wauters A, Franck F, Daelemans R, & Neels H (1994) Excess serum osmolality gap after ingestion of methanol: A methodology-associated phenomenon? Clin Chem, **40**: 1587-1590.

Dethlefs R & Naraqi S (1978) Ocular manifestations and complications of acute methyl alcohol intoxication. Med J Aust, **2**: 483-485.

Diaz-Rueda J, Sloane HJ, & Obremski RJ (1977) An infrared solution method for the analysis of trapped atmospheric contaminants desorbed from charcoal tubes. Appl Spectrom, **31**: 298-307.

Donnelly MI & Dagley S (1980) Production of methanol from amino acids by *Pseudomonas putida*. J Bacteriol, **142**: 916-924.

Dorman DC, Dye JA, Nassise MP, Ekuta J, Bolon B, & Medinsky MA (1993) Acute methanol toxicity in minipigs. Fundam Appl Toxicol, **20**: 341-347.

Dorman DC, Moss OR, Farris GM, Janszen D, Bond JA, & Medinsky MA (1994) Pharmacokinetics of inhaled ^{14}C-methanol and methanol-derived ^{14}C-formate in normal and folate-deficient cynomologus monkeys. Toxicol Appl Pharmacol, **128**: 229-238.

Dorman DC, Bolon B, Struve MF, La Perle KMD, Wong BA, Elswick BE, & Welsch F (1995) Role of formate in methanol-induced exencephaly. Teratology, **52**: 30-40.

Dowling JE (1987) The electroretinogram and glial responses. In: Dowling JE ed. The retina: An approachable part of the brain. Cambridge, Massachusetts, Belknapp Press, pp 164-186.

Downie A, Khattab TM, Malik IA, & Samara IN (1992) A case of percutaneous industrial methanol toxicity. Occup Med, **42**: 47-49.

Dube MF & Green CR (1982) Methods of collection of smoke for analytical purposes. Recent Adv Tob Sci, **8**: 42-102.

Dutkiewicz B, Konczalik J, & Karwacki W (1980) Skin absorption and per os administration of methanol in men. Int Arch Occup Environ Health, **47**: 81-88.

Ebron-McCoy MT, Andrews JE, Kavlock RJ, & Rogers LM (1994) The developmental toxicity of formate and formic acid in mouse and rat embryos in whole culture (WEC). Teratology, **49**: 393.

Eells JT (1991) Methanol- induced visual toxicity in the rat. J Pharmacol Exp Ther, **257**: 56-63.

Eells JT, Makar AB, Noker PE, & Tephly TR (1981a) Methanol poisoning and formate oxidation in nitrous oxide-treated rats. J Pharmacol Exp Ther, **217**: 57-61.

Eells JT, McMartin KE, Black K, Virayotha V, Tisdell RH, & Tephly TR (1981b) Formaldehyde poisoning: a rapid metabolism to formic acid. J Am Med Assoc, **246**: 1237-1238.

Eells JT, Black KA, Makar AB, Tedford CE, & Tephly TR (1982) The regulation of one-carbon oxidation in the rat by nitrous oxide and methionine. Arch Biochem Biophys, **219**: 316-326.

Eells JT, Black KA, Tedford CE, & Tephly TR (1983) Methanol toxicity in the monkey: effects of nitrous oxide and methionine. J Pharmacol Exp Ther, **227**: 349-353.

Eells JT, Salzman MM, & Trusk TC (1995) Inhibition of retinal mitochondrial function in methanol intoxication. Toxicologist, **15**: 21-23.

Eells JT, Salzman MM, Lewandowski MF, & Murray TG (1996) Formate induced alterations in retinal function in methanol-intoxicated rats. Toxicol Appl Pharmacol, **140**: 58-69.

Eells JT, Salzman MM, Lewandowski MF, & Murray TG (in press) Developmental and characterization of a non-primate animal model of methanol induced neurotoxicity. In: Bengston DA & Henschel DS ed. Environmental toxicology and risk assessment: Biomarkers and risk assessment - Volume 5. Philadelphia, Pennsylvania, American Society for Testing and Materials, (Publication ASTM STP No. 1306).

Egle JL & Gochberg BJ (1979) Retention of inhaled isoprene and methanol in the dog. Am Ind Hyg Assoc J, **36**: 369-373.

Eisenberg AA (1917) Visceral changes in wood alcohol poisoning by inhalation. Am J Public Health, **7**: 765-771.

Eisenreich SJ, Looney BB, & Thornton JD (1981) Airborne organic contaminants in the Great Lakes ecosystem. Environ Sci Technol, **15**: 30-38.

Elvers B, Hawkins S, & Schulz G ed. (1990) Ullmann's encyclopedia of industrial chemistry, 5th ed. Weinheim, Germany, VCH-Verlag, vol 16A, pp 465-486.

Eriksen SP & Kulkarni AB (1963) Methanol in normal human breath. Science, **141**: 639-640.

Erlanson P, Fritz H, Hagstam KE, Liljenberg B, Tryding N, & Voigt G (1965) Severe methanol intoxication. Acta Med Scand, **177**: 393-408.

Ewell WS, Gorsuch JW, Kringle RO, Robillard KA, & Spiegel RC (1986) Simultaneous evolution of the acute effects of chemicals on seven aquatic species. Environ Toxicol Chem, **5**: 831-840.

FAO/WHO (1971) Toxicological evaluation of some extraction solvents and certain other substances. Report of the Joint FAO/WHO Expert Committee on Food Additives, 24 June-2 July 1970. Rome, Food and Agriculture Organization, pp 105-109.

Federal Register (1989) Standards for emissions from methanol-fueled motor vehicles and motor vehicle engines - Final rule. Fed Reg, **54**(68): 40CFR Part 86.

Feldstein M & Klendshoj RE (1954) Determination of methanol in biological fluids by microdiffusion analysis. Anal Chem, **26**: 932-933.

Ferry DG, Temple WA, & McQueen EG (1980) Methanol monitoring. Int Arch Occup Environ Health, **47**: 155-163.

Fiedler E, Grossmann G, Kersebohm B, Weiss G, & Witte C (1990) Methanol. In: Elvers B, Hawkins S, & Schutz G ed. Ullmann's encyclopedia of industrial chemistry, 5th ed. Weinheim, VCH Verlagsgesellschaft, vol 16A, pp 465-486.

Filley CM & Kelly JP (1993) Alcohol-and drug-related neurotoxicity. Current Opin Neurol Neurosurg, **6**: 443-447.

Fox ME (1973) Rapid gas chromatographic method for determination of residual methanol in sewage. Environ Sci Technol, **7**: 838-840.

Francot P & Geoffroy P (1956) Le méthanol dans les jus de fruits, les boissons fermentées des alcools et spiriteux. Rev Ferment Ind Aliment, **11**: 279-287.

Franzblau A, Levine SP, Burgess LA, Qu QS, Schreck RM, & D'Arcy JB (1992a) The use of a transportable Fourier Transform infrared (FTIR) spectrometer for the direct measurement of solvents in breath and ambient air: I. Methanol. Am Ind Hyg Assoc J, **53**: 221-227.

Franzblau A, Levine SP, D'Arcy JB, & Qu QS (1992b) Use of urinary formic acid as a biologic exposure index of methanol exposure. Appl Occup Environ Hyg, **7**: 467-471.

Franzblau A, Lee EW, Schreck RM, D'Arcy JB, Santrock J, & Levine SP (1993) Absence of formic acid accumulation in urine following five days of methanol exposure. Appl Occup Environ Hyg, **8**: 883-888.

Frederick LJ, Schulte PA, & Apol A (1984) Investigation and control of occupational hazards associated with the use of spirit duplicators. Am Ind Hyg Assoc J, **45**: 51-55.

Freitag D, Ballhorn L, Geyer H, & Korte F (1985) Environmental hazard profile of organic chemicals. Chemosphere, **14**: 1589-1616.

Frenia MI & Schauben JL (1993) Methanol inhalation toxicity. Ann Emerg Med, **22**: 1919-1923.

Gabele PA & Knapp KT (1993) A characterization of emissions from an early model flexible-fuel vehicle. J Air Waste Manage Assoc, **43**: 851-858.

Garcia JH & Van Zandt JP (1969) Proceedings of 27th Annual Meeting of the Electron Microscope Society of America. Baton Rouge, Louisiana, Claitor Publishers, vol 27, pp 360-361.

Garner CD & Lee EW (1994) Evaluation of methanol-induced retinotoxicity using oscillatory potential analysis. Toxicology, **93**: 113-124.

Garner CD, Lee EW, & Louis-Ferdinand RJ (1995a) Muller cell involvement in methanol-induced retinal toxicity. Toxicol Appl Pharmacol, **130**: 101-107.

Garner CD, Lee EW, Terzo TS, & Louis-Ferdinand RJ (1995b) The role of retinal metabolism in methanol-induced retinal toxicity. J Toxicol Environ Health, **44**: 43-56.

Gessner PK (1970) Method for the assay of ethanol and other aliphatic alcohols applicable to tissue homogenates and possessing a sensitivity of 1 μg/ml. Anal Biochem, **38**: 499-505.

Gettler AO (1920) Critical study of methods for the detection of methyl alcohol. J Biol Chem, **42**: 311-328.

Geyer H, Politzki G, & Freitag D (1984) Prediction of ecological behavior of chemicals: relationship between n-octanol/water partition and bioaccumulation of organic chemicals by alga Chlorella. Chemosphere, **13**: 269-284.

Gilger AP & Potts AM (1955) Studies on the visual toxicity of methanol: V. The role of acidosis in experimental methanol poisoning. Am J Ophthamol, **39**: 63-86.

Gilger AP, Potts AM, & Johnson JV (1952) Studies on the visual toxicity of methanol: II. The effect of parenterally administered substances on the systemic toxicity of methyl alcohol. Am J Ophthamol, **35**(Part 2): 113-126.

Giminez ER, Vallejo NE, Roy E, Lis M, Izurieta EM, Rossi S, & Capuccio M (1968) Percutaneous alcohol intoxication. Clin Toxicol, **1**: 39-48.

Glazer M & Dross P (1993) Necrosis of the putamen caused by methanol intoxication: MR findings. Am J Roentgenol, **160**: 1105-1106.

Gluth G & Hanke W (1985) A comparison of physiological changes in carp, *Cyprinus carpio*, induced by several pollutants at sublethal concentrations: 1. The dependency on exposure times. Ecotoxicol Environ Saf, **9**: 179-188.

Gluth G, Freitag D, Hanke W, & Korte F (1985) Accumulation of pollutants in fish. Comp Biochem Physiol, **81C**: 273-277.

Gold MD & Moulif CE (1988) Effects of emission standards on methanol vehicle-related ozone, formaldehyde and methanol exposure. Presented at 81st Meeting of Air Pollution Control Association, Dallas, TX, June 19-24. Pittsburgh, Pennsylvania, Air Pollution Control Association.

Gonda A, Gault H, Churchill D, & Hollomby D (1978) Hemodialysis for methanol intoxication. Am J Med, **64**: 749-757.

Goodman JI & Tephly TR (1971) A comparison of rat and human liver formaldehyde dehydrogenase. Biochim Biophys Acta, **252**: 489.

Grady S & Osterloh J (1986) Improved enzymic assay for serum formate with colorimetric endpoint. J Anal Toxicol, **10**: 1-5.

Graedel TE, Hawkins DT, & Claxton LD ed. (1986) Atmospheric chemical compounds: Sources, occurrence and bioassay. New York, London, Academic Press, pp 512-514, 557.

Grayson M ed. (1981) Kirk-Othmer encyclopedia of chemical technology, 3rd ed. New York, John Wiley & Son, vol 15, pp 398-405.

Greenberg L, Mayers MR, Goldwater LJ, & Burke WJ (1938) Health hazards in the manufacture of "fused collars": II. Exposure to acetone-methanol. J Ind Hyg Toxicol, **20**: 148-154.

Greizerstein HB (1981) Congener contents of alcoholic beverages. J Stud Alcohol, **42**: 1030-1037.

Griffiths AJF (1981) Neurospora and environmentally induced aneuploidy. In: Stich HF & San RHC ed. Short-term tests for chemical carcinogens. Berlin, Heidelberg, New York, Springer-Verlag, pp 187-199.

Guerin MR, Higgins CE, & Greist WH (1987) The analysis of the particulate and vapour phases of tobacco smoke. In: O'Neill IK, Brunnemann KD, Dodet B, & Hoffmann D ed. Environmental carcinogens: Methods of analysis and exposure measurement, Volume 9. Lyon, International Agency for Research on Cancer, pp 115-139 (IARC Scientific Publications No. 81).

Guggenheim MA, Couch JR, & Weinberg W (1971) Motor dysfunction as a permanent complication of methanol ingestion. Arch Neurol, **24**: 550-554.

Güsten H, Klasinc L, & Maric D (1984) Prediction of the abiotic degradability of organic compounds in the troposphere. J Atmos Chem, **2**: 83-93.

Haggard HW & Greenberg LA (1939) Studies on the absorption, distribution and elimination of alcohol: IV. The elimination of methylalcohol. J Pharmacol Exp Ther, **66**: 479-496.

Hanson RS (1980) Ecology and diversity of methylotropic organisms. Adv Appl Microbiol, **26**: 3-29.

Harger RN (1935) A simple micromethod for the determination of alcohol in biological material. J Lab Clin Med, **20**: 746-751.

Hatfield R (1957) Biological oxidation of some organic compounds. Ind Eng Chem, **49**: 192-197.

Hayreh MS, Hayreh SS, Baumbach GL, Cancilla P, Martin-Amat G, Tephly TR, McMartin KE, & Makar AB (1977) Methyl alcohol poisoning: III. Ocular toxicity. Arch Ophthamol, **95**: 1851-1858.

Heath A (1983) Methanol poisoning. Lancet, 1: 1339-1340.

Heath M (1991) Alternative transportation fuels: Natural gas, propane, methanol and ethanol compared with gasoline and diesel. Calgary, Canadian Energy Research Institute, pp 113-115.

HEI (1987) Automotive methanol vapors and human health: An evaluation of existing scientific information and issues for future research. Cambridge, Massachusetts, Health Effects Institute, 70 pp (Special Report).

HEI (1996) The potential health effects of oxygenates added to gasoline: A review of the current literature. Cambridge, Massachusetts, Health Effects Institute, 165 pp.

Heidelberger C, Freeman AE, Pienta RJ, Sivak A, Bertram DS, Casto BC, & Dunkel VC (1983) Cell transformation by chemical agents: A review and analysis of the literature. Mutat Res, **114**: 283-385.

Heinrich R & Angerer J (1982) Occupational chronic exposure to organic solvents. Int Arch Occup Environ Health, **50**: 341-349.

Helmstetter A, Gamerdinger AP, & Pruell RJ (1996) Acute toxicity of methanol to *Mytilus edulis*. Bull Environ Contam Toxicol, **57**(4): 675-681.

Hemming DJB, Criddle RS, & Hansen LD (1995) Effects of methanol on plant respiration. J Plant Physiol, **146**(3): 193-198.

Hermens J & Leeuwangh P (1982) Joint toxicity of mixtures of 8 and 24 chemicals to the guppy (*Poecilia reticulata*) Ecotoxicol Environ Saf, **6**: 302-310.

Hertelendy ZI, Mendenhall CL, Rouster SD, Marshall L, & Weesner R (1993) Biochemical and clinical effects of aspartame in patients with chronic, stable alcoholic liver disease. Am J Gastroenterol, **88**: 737-743.

Hickman GT & Novak JT (1989) Relationship between subsurface biodegradation rates and microbial density. Environ Sci Technol, **23**: 525-532.

Hickman GT, Novak JT, Morris MS, & Rebhun M (1989) Effects of site variations on subsurface biodegradation potential. J Water Pollut Control Fed, **61**: 1564-1575.

Hindberg J & Wieth JO (1963) Quantitative determination of methanol in biological fluids. J Lab Clin Med, **61**: 355-361.

Hippe H, Caspari D, Fiebig K, & Gottschalk G (1979) Utilization of trimethylamine and other N-methyl compounds for growth and methane formation by methanosarcina barkeri. Proc Natl Acad Sci (USA), **76**: 494-498.

Holzer G, Shanfield H, Zlatkis A, Bertsch W, Juarez P, Mayfield H, & Liebich HM (1977) Collection and analysis of trace emissions from natural sources. J Chromatogr, **142**: 755-764.

Hooper AB & Terry KR (1973) Specific inhibitors of ammonia oxidation in Nitrosomonas. J Bacteriol, **115**: 480-485.

Horton VI, Higuchi MA, & Rickert DE (1992) Physiologically based pharmacokinetic model for methanol in rats, monkeys and humans. Toxicol Appl Pharmacol, **117**: 26-36.

Howard PH ed. (1990) Handbook of environmental fate and exposure data for organic compounds - Volume II: Solvents. Chelsea, Michigan, Lewis Publishers, pp 310-317.

Howard PH, Boethling RS, Jarvis WF, Meylan WM, & Michalenko EM (1991) Handbook of environmental degradation rates. Chelsea, Michigan, Lewis Publishers, pp 93-94.

Hsieh FY, Leu TM, & Chia LG (1992) Bilateral putaminal necrosis caused by methanol poisoning: A case report. Chin Med J (Taipei), **49**: 283-288.

Hüls AG (1978) [Determination of the biodegradability of methanol in the closed bootle tert (OECD Guideline 30D).] Marl, Hüls AG, 11 pp (in German).

Hunt R (1902) The toxicity of methyl alcohol. John Hopkins Hosp Bull, **13**: 213.

Hustert K, Mansour M, Parlar H, & Korte F (1981) [The EPA test - A method for the determination of photochemical degradation of organic compounds in aquatic systems.] Chemosphere, **10**: 995-998 (in German).

ILO (1983) In: Parmeggiani L ed. Encyclopedia of occupational health and safety, 3rd revis ed. Geneva, International Labour Office, vol 2, pp 1356-1358.

ILO (1991) Occupational exposure limits for airborne toxic substances, 3rd ed. Geneva, International Labour Office, pp 256-257.

Infurna R & Weiss B (1986) Neonatal behavioural toxicity in rats following prenatal exposures to methanol. Teratology, **33**: 259-265.

Ingemansson SO (1983) Studies on the effect of 4-methylpyrazole on retinal activity in the methanol poisoned monkey by recording the electroretinogram. Acta Opthalmol, **158**(Suppl): 5-24.

IPCS (1995) Poison Information Monograph No. 335: Methanol. Geneva, World Health Organization, International Programme on Chemical Safety.

Isidorov VA, Zenkevich IG, & Ioffe BV (1985) Volatile organic compounds in the atmosphere of forests. Atmos Environ, **19**: 1-8.

Jacobs GA (1990) OECD eye irritation tests on three alcohols; Acute toxicity data. J Am Coll Toxicol, **1**: 56-57.

Jacobsen D & McMartin KE (1986) Methanol and ethylene glycol poisonings: Mechanisms of toxicity, clinical course, diagnosis and treatment. Med Toxicol, **1**: 309-314.

Jacobsen D, Jansen H, Wiek-Larsen E, Bredesen DE, & Halvorsen S (1982a) Studies on methanol poisoning. Acta Med Scand, **12**: 5-10.

Jacobsen D, Bredesen JE, Eide I, & Ostborg J (1982b) Anion and osmolal gaps in the diagnosis of methanol and ethylene glycol poisoning. Acta Med Scand, **212**: 17-20.

Jacobsen D, Ovrebo S, & Sejersted OM (1983a) Toxicokinetics of formate during hemodialysis. Acta Med Scand, **214**: 409-412.

Jacobsen D, Ovrebo S, Arnesen E, & Paus PN (1983b) Pulmonary excretion of methanol in man. Scand J Clin Invest, **43**: 377-379.

Jacobsen D, Webb P, Collins TD, & McMartin KE (1988) Methanol and formate kinetics in late diagnosed methanol intoxication. Med Toxicol, **3**: 418-423.

Jacobsen D, Sebastian CS, Barron SK, Carriere EW, & McMartin KE (1990) Effects of 4-methylpyrazole, methanol/ethylene glycol antidote in healthy humans. J Emerg Med, **8**: 455-461.

Jansen JLC, Nyberg U, Aspegren H, & Andersson B (1993) Handling of anaerobic digester supernatant combined with full nitrogen removal. Water Sci Technol, **27**: 391-403.

Jaselkis B & Warriner JP (1966) Titrimetric determination of primary and secondary alcohols by xenon trioxide oxidation. Anal Chem, **38**: 563-564.

Jeganathan PS & Namasivayam A (1989) Methanol induced monoamine changes in hypothalamus and striatum of albino rats. Alcohol, **6**: 451-454.

Jones AW (1986) Abnormally high concentrations of methanol in breath: A useful biochemical marker of recent heavy drinking. Clin Chem, **32**: 1241-1242.

Jones AW (1987) Elimination half-life of methanol during hangover. Pharmacol Toxicol, **60**: 217-220.

Jones AW & Lowinger H (1988) Relationship between the concentration of ethanol and methanol in blood samples from Swedish drinking drivers. Forensic Sci Int, **37**: 277-285.

Jones AW, Mardh G, & Anggard E (1983) Determination and endogenous ethanol in blood and breath by gas chromatography-mass spectrometry. Pharmacol Biochem Behav, **18**(Suppl 1): 267-272.

Jones AW, Skagerberg S, Yonekurat T, & Sato A (1990) Metabolic interaction between endogenous ethanol studied in human volunteers by analysis of breath. Pharmacol Toxicol, **66**: 62-65.

Jonsson A & Berg S (1983) Determination of low-molecular-weight oxygenated hydrocarbons in ambient air by cryogradient sampling and two-dimensional gas chromatography. J Chromatogr, **279**: 307-322.

Jonsson A, Persson KA, & Grigoriadis V (1985) Measurements of some low molecular-weight oxygenated, aromatic and chlorinated hydrocarbons in ambient air and in vehicle emissions. Environ Int, **11**: 383-392.

Juhnke VI & Lüdemann D (1978) [Results of testing of 200 chemical compounds for acute fish toxicity with the Golden Orfe test.] Z Wasser Abwasser Forsch, **11**(5): 161-164 (in German).

Jungclaus GA, Lopez-Avila V, & Hites RA (1978) Organic compounds in an industrial wastewater: A case study of their environmental impact. Environ Sci Technol, **12**: 88-96.

Kahn A & Blum D (1979) Methyl alcohol poisoning in an 8-month old boy: An unusual rank route of intoxication. J Pediatr, **94**: 841-843.

Kane RI, Talbert W, Harlan J, Sizemore G, & Cataland S (1968) A methanol poisoning outbreak in Kentucky. Arch Environ Health, **17**: 119-129.

Kaplan K (1962) Methyl alcohol poisoning. Am J Med Sci, **244**: 170-174.

Katoh M (1989) New Energy Development Organization data. Presented at the Methanol Vapors and Health Effects Workshop: What we know and what we need to know - Summary Report. Washington, DC, ILSI Risk Science Institute/US Environmental Protection Agency/Health Effects Institute/American Petroleum Institute, p A-7.

Kavet R & Nauss KM (1990) The toxicity of inhaled methanol vapors. CRC Crit Rev Toxicol, **21**: 21-50.

Kawai T, Yasugi T, Uchida Y, & Ikeda M (1990) Personal diffusive sampler for methanol, a hydrophilic solvent. Bull Environ Contam Toxicol, **44**: 514-520.

Kawai T, Yasugi T, Mizunuma K, Horiguchi S, Hirase Y, Uchida Y, & Ikeda M (1991a) Simple method for the determination of methanol in blood and its application in occupational health. Bull Environ Contam Toxicol, **47**: 797-803.

Kawai T, Yasugi T, Mizunuma K, Horiguchi S, Hirase Y, Uchida Y, & Ikeda M (1991b) Methanol in urine as a biological indicator of occupational exposure to methanol vapor. Int Arch Occup Environ Health, **63**: 311-318.

Kawai T, Yasugi T, Mizunuma K, Horiguchi S, Iguchi H, Uchida Y, Iwami O, & Ikeda m (1992) Comparative evaluation of urinalysis and blood analysis as means of detecting exposure to organic solvents at low concentrations. Int Arch Occup Environ Health, **64**: 223-234.

Kawai T, Mizunuma K, Yasugi T, Horiguchi S, Moon CS, Zhang ZW, Miyashita K, Takeda S, & Ikeda M (1995) Effects of methanol on styrene metabolism among workers occupationally exposed at low concentrations. Arch Environ Contam Toxicol, **28**: 543-546.

Keeney AH & Mellinkoff SM (1951) Methyl alcohol poisoning. Ann Intern Med, **34**: 331-338.

Keller AE (1993) Acute toxicity of several pesticides, organic compounds, and a wastewater effluent to the fresh water mussel, Anodonta imbecilis, *Ceriodaphnia dubia* and *Pimephales promelas*. Bull Environ Contam Toxicol, **51**: 696-702.

Kelly TJ, Mukund R, Spicer CW, & Pollack AJ (1994) Concentrations and transformations of hazardous air pollutants. Environ Sci Technol, **28**: 378A-387A.

Kennedy TF & Shanks D (1981) Methanol: manufacture and uses. In: Wickson EJ ed. Monohydric alcohols. Washington, DC, American Chemical Society, pp 19-27 (ACS Symposium Series No. 159).

Kempa ES (1976) [Oxygen needs during the degradation of waste compounds.] Österr Abwasser Rundsch, **2**: 20-25 (in German).

Keyvan-Larijarni H & Tannenberg AM (1974) Methanol intoxication: Comparison of peritoneal dialysis and hemodialysis treatment. Arch Intern Med, **124**: 293-296.

Kim S (1973) Purification and properties of protein methylase. Arch Biochem Biophys, **157**: 476-484.

Kimura ET, Ebert DM, & Dodge PW (1971) Acute toxicity and limits of solvent residue for sixteen organic solvents. Toxicol Appl Pharmacol, **19**: 699-704.

King L (1992) Acute methanol poisoning: A case study. Heart Lung, **21**: 260-264.

King GM, Klug MJ, & Lovley DR (1983) Metabolism of acetate, methanol and methylated amines in intertidal sediments of Lowes Cove, Maine. Appl Environ Microbiol, **45**: 1848-1853.

Kingsley WH & Hirsch FG (1955) Toxicological considerations in direct process spirit duplicating machines. Compens Med, **6**: 7-8.

Kinlin TE, Muralidhara R, Pittet AO, Sanderson A, & Walradt JP (1972) Volatile components of roasted filberts. J Agric Food Chem, **20**: 1021-1028.

Kinoshita JH & Masurat T (1958) Effect of glutathione in formaldehyde oxidation in the retina. Am J Opthalmol, **46**: 42.

Kirchner JG & Miller JM (1957) Volatile water-soluble and oil constituents of Valencia orange juice. J Agric Food Chem, **5**: 283-291.

Kohl WL ed. (1990) Methanol as an alternative fuel choice: An assessment. Washington, DC, The Johns Hopkins University School of Foreign Service, pp 439.

Koivusalo M (1970) Methanol. In: Tremolieres J ed. International encyclopaedia of pharmacology and therapeutics. Oxford, New York, Pergamon Press, vol 2, section 20, pp 465-505.

Komers R & Sir Z (1976) Gas chromatographic determination at the parts per million level of methanol and ethanol in aqueous solution. J Chromatogr, **119**: 251-254.

Konemann H (1981) Quantitative structure-activity relationships in fish toxicity studies. Toxicology, **19**: 209-221.

Krotoszynski B, Gabriel G, O'Neill HJ, & Claudio MPA (1977) Characterization of human expired air: A promising investigative and diagnostic technique. J Chromatogr Sci, **15**: 239-244.

Krotoszynski BK, Bruneau GM, & O'Neill HJ (1979) Measurement of chemical inhalation exposure in urban populations in the presence of endogenous effluents. J Anal Toxicol, **3**: 225-234.

Kruse JA (1992) Methanol poisoning. Intensive Care Med, **18**: 391-397.

Kuhn R, Pattard M, Pernak KD, & Winter A (1989) Results of the harmful effects of selected water pollutants (anilines, phenols, aliphatic compounds) to *Daphnia magna*. Water Res, **23**: 495-499.

Kutzbach C & Stokstad ELR (1968) Partial purification of a 10-formyl tetrahydrofolate: NADP oxidoreductase from mammalian liver. Biochem Biophys Res Commun, **30**: 111.

Larsson BT (1965) Gas chromatography of organic volatiles in human breath and saliva. Acta Med Scand, **19**: 159-164.

Leaf G & Zatman LJ (1952) A study of the conditions under which methanol may exert a toxic hazard in industry. Br J Ind Med, **9**: 19-31.

Lee EW, Reader JA, Garner CD, Brady AN, & Li LC (1990) Evaluation of methanol (M) toxicity on the visual system: spontaneous degeneration of the retina and optic nerve in the F-344 rat. Toxicologist, **10**: 155.

Lee EW, Brady AN, Brabec MJ, & Fabelt JN (1991) Effects of methanol vapors on testosterone production and testis morphology in rats. Toxicol Ind Health, **7**: 261-275.

Lee EW, Terzo TS, D'Arcy JB, Gross KB, & Schreck RM (1992) Lack of blood formate accumulation in humans following exposure to methanol vapors at the current permissible exposure limit of 200 ppm. Am Ind Hyg Assoc J, **53**: 99-104.

Lee EW, Garner CD, & Terzo TS (1994a) Animal model for the study of methanol toxicity: Comparison of folate-reduced rat responses with published monkey data. J Toxicol Environ Health, **41**: 71-82.

Lee EW, Garner CD, & Terzo TS (1994b) A rat model manifesting methanol-induced visual dysfunction suitable for both acute and long-term exposure studies. Toxicol Appl Pharmacol, **128**: 199-206.

Lemaire J, Campbell I, Hulpke H, Guth JA, Merz W, Philp J, & von Waldow C (1982) An assessment of test methods for photodegradation of chemicals in the environment. Chemosphere, **11**: 119-164.

Lettinga G, De Zeeuw W, & Ouberg E (1981) Anaerobic treatment of wastes containing methanol and higher alcohols. Water Res, **15**: 171-182.

Lewis RJ Sr (1989) Food additives handbook. New York, Van Nostrand Reinhold Co., pp 291-292.

Ley CO & Gali FG (1983) Parkinsonian syndrome after methanol intoxication. Eur Neurol, **22**: 405-409.

Liesivuori J & Savolainen H (1987) Urinary formic acid as an indicator of occupational exposure to formic acid and methanol. Am Ind Hyg Assoc J, **48**: 32-34.

Liesivuori J & Savolainen H (1991) Methanol and formic acid toxicity: Biochemical mechanisms. Pharmacol Toxicol, **69**: 157-163.

Lijinsky W, Thomas BJ, & Kovatch RM (1991) Differences in skin carcinogenesis by methyl nitroso urea between mice of several strains. Cancer Lett, **61**: 1-5.

Linden E, Bengtsson BE, Svanberg O, & Sundstrom G (1979) The acute toxicity of 78 chemicals and pesticide formulations against two brackish water organisms - The bleak (*Alburnus alburnus*) and the harpacticoid nitocraspinipes. Chemosphere, **11/12**: 843-851.

Lins RL, Zachee P, Christiaens M, Van De Vijver F, De Waele L, Sandra P, & De Broe ME (1980) Prognosis and treatment of methanol intoxication. In: Holmstedt B, Lauwerys R, Mercier M, & Roberfroid M ed. Mechanisms of toxicity and hazard evaluation. Amsterdam, Elsevier/North-Holland Biomedical Press, pp 415-421.

Litovitz LT, Schmitz BF, Matyunas N, & Martin TG (1988) 1987 Annual report of the American Association of Poison Control Centers National Data Collection System. Am J Emerg Med, **6**: 479-515.

Loewy A & von der Heide R (1914) [The uptake of methyl alcohol by inhalation.] Biochem Ztg, **65**: 230-252 (in German).

Løkke H (1984) Leaching of ethylene glycol and ethanol in subsoils. Water Air Soil Pollut, **22**: 373-387.

Lovegren NV, Fisher GS, Legendre MG, & Schuller WH (1979) Volatile constituents of dried legumes. J Agric Food Chem, **27**: 851-853.

Luke LA & Ray JE (1984) Gas-chromatographic method for the determination of low relative molecular mass alcohols and methyl tert-butyl ether in gasoline. Analyst, **109**: 989-992.

Lund A (1948a) Excretion of methanol and formic acid in man after methanol consumption. Acta Pharmacol, **4**: 205-212.

Lund A (1948b) Metabolism of methanol and formic acid in dogs. Acta Pharmacol, **4**: 108-121.

Lund A (1948c) Metabolism of methanol and formic acid in rabbits. Acta Pharmacol, **4**: 99-107.

Lund ED, Kirkland CL, & Shaw PE (1981) Methanol, ethanol and acetaldehyde contents of citrus products. J Agric Food Chem, **29**: 361-366.

Lundberg P (1985) Scientific basis for Swedish occupational standards VI. Arb Och Halsa, **32**: 115-121.

Lyman WJ, Reehl WF, & Rosenblatt DH ed. (1990) Handbook of chemical property estimation methods. Washington, DC, American Chemical Society.

McCord CP (1931) Toxicity of methyl alcohol (methanol) following skin absorption and inhalation. Ind Eng Chem, **23**: 931-936.

McCoy H, Cipolle RJ, Ehlers SM, Sawchuk RJ, & Zaske DE (1979) Severe methanol poisoning: Application of a pharmacokinetic model for ethanol therapy and hemodialysis. Am J Med, **67**: 804-807.

McDonald A, Sey YM, House DE, & Simmons JE (1992) Methanol potentiation of carbon tetrachloride hepatotoxicity is dependent on the time of carbon tetrachloride administration. Toxicologist, **12**: 239.

McGregor DB, Martin R, Riach CG, & Caspary WJ (1985) Optimization of a metabolic activation system for use in the mouse lymphoma L5178Y tk$^+$tk- mutation system. Environ Mutagen, **7**(Suppl 3): 10.

Machiele PA (1990) A health and safety assessment of methanol as an alternative fuel. In: Kohl WL ed. Methanol as an alternative choice. Washington, DC, The Johns Hopkins Foreign Policy Institute, pp 217-239.

McLean DR, Jacobs H, & Mielke BW (1980) Methanol poisoning: A clinical and pathological study. Ann Neurol, **8**: 162-167.

McMartin KE, Makar AB, Martin-Amat G, Palese M, & Tephly TR (1975) Methanol poisoning I. The role of formic acid in the development of metabolic acidosis in the monkey and the reversal by 4-methylpyrazole. Biochem Med, **13**: 319-333.

McMartin KE, Martin-Amat G, Makar AB, & Tephly TR (1977) Methanol poisoning: V. The role of formate metabolism in the monkey. J Pharmacol Exp Ther, **201**: 564-572.

McMartin KE, Martin-Amat G, Noker PE, & Tephly TR (1979) Lack of a role for formaldehyde in methanol poisoning in the monkey. Biochem Pharmacol, **28**: 645-649.

McMartin KE, Ambre JJ, & Tephly TR (1980a) Methanol poisoning in human subjects: Role of formic acid accumulation in the metabolic acidosis. Am J Med, **68**: 414-418.

McMartin KE, Hedstrom KG, Tolf BR, Ostung-Wintzell H, & Blomstrand R (1980b) Studies on the metabolic interactions between 4-methylpyrazole and methanol using the monkey as an animal model. Arch Biochem Biophys, **199**: 606-614.

Maeda Y, Fujio Y, Suetaka T, & Munemori M (1988) Selective gas chromatographic determination of trace amounts of alcohols in ambient air. Analyst, **113**: 189-191.

Maejima K, Suzuki T, Niwa H, Maekawa A, Nagase S, & Ishinishi N (1992) Toxicity to rats of methanol-fueled engine exhaust continuously for 28 days. J Toxicol Environ Health, **37**: 293-312.

Maejima K, Suzuki T, Numata H, Maekawa A, Nagase S, & Ishinishi N (1993) Recovery from changes in the blood and nasal cavity and/or lungs of rats caused by exposure to methanol-fueled engine exhaust. J Toxicol Environ Health, **39**: 323-340.

Maejima K, Suzuki T, Numata H, Maekawa A, Nagase S, & Ishinishi N (1994) Subchronic (12-week) inhalation toxicity study of methanol-fueled engine exhaust in rats. J Toxicol Environ Health, **41**: 315-327.

Mahieu P, Hassoun A, & Lauwerys R (1989) Predictors of methanol intoxication with unfavourable outcome. Hum Toxicol, **8**: 135-137.

Majchrowicz E & Mendelson JH (1971) Blood methanol concentrations during experimentally induced ethanol intoxication in alcoholics. J Pharmacol Exp Ther, **179**: 293-300.

Makar AB & Mannering GJ (1968) Role of the intracellular distribution of hepatic catalase in the peroxidative oxidation of methanol. Mol Pharmacol, **4**: 484-491.

Makar AB & Tephly TR (1976) Methanol poisoning in the folate deficient rat. Nature (Lond), **261**: 715-716.

Makar AB & Tephly TR (1977) Methanol poisoning: VI. Role of folic acid in the production of methanol poisoning in the rat. J Toxicol Environ Health, **2**: 1201-1209.

Makar AB & Tephly TR (1982) Improved estimation of formate in body fluids and tissues. Clin Chem, **28**: 385.

Makar AB, Tephly TR, & Mannering GJ (1968) Methanol metabolism in the monkey. Mol Pharmacol, **4**: 471-483.

Makar AB, McMartin KE, Palese M, & Tephly TR (1975) Formate assay in body fluids: application to methanol poisoning. Biochem Med, **13**: 117-126.

Makar AB, Tephly TR, Sahin G, & Osweiler G (1990) Formate metabolism in young swine. Toxicol Appl Pharmacol, **105**: 315-320.

Malorny G, Rietbrock N, & Schneider M (1965) [The oxidation of formaldehyde to formic acid in blood: a contribution to the metabolism of formaldehyde.] Naunyn Schmiedebergs Arch Pathol Exp Pharmacol, **250**: 419-436 (in German).

Martin-Amat G, Tephly TR, McMartin KE, Makar AB, Hayreh MS, Hayreh SS, Baumbach G, & Cancilla P (1977) Methyl alcohol poisoning: II. Development of a model for ocular toxicity in methyl alcohol poisoning using the rhesus monkey. Arch Ophthamol, **95**: 1847-1850.

Martin-Amat G, McMartin KE, Hayreh SS, & Tephly TR (1978) Methanol poisoning: Ocular toxicity produced by formate. Toxicol Appl Pharmacol, **45**: 201-208.

Martinasevic MK, Green MD, Baron J, & Tephly TR (1996) Folate and 10 formyltetrahydrofolate dehydrogenase in human and rat retina: relation to methanol toxicity. Toxicol Appl Pharmacol, **141**: 373-381.

Mashbitz LM, Sklianskaya RM, & Urieva FI (1936) The relative toxicity of acetone, methyl alcohol and their mixtures: II. Their action on white mice. J Ind Hyg Toxicol, **18**: 117-122.

Mather A & Assimos A (1965) Evaluation of gas-liquid chromatography in assays for blood volatiles. Clin Chem, **11**: 1023-1035.

Matsui S, Okawa Y, & Ota R (1988) Experience of 16 years' operation and maintenance of the Fukashiba industrial wastewater treatment plant of the Kashima petrochemical complex: II. Biodegradability of 37 organic substances and 28 process waste waters. Water Sci Technol, **20**: 201-210.

Mayer FL & Ellersieck MR (1986) Manual of acute toxicity: Interpretation and database for 410 chemicals and 66 species of freshwater animals. Washington, DC, US Department of the Interior, Fish and Wildlife Service (Resource Publication No. 160).

Medinsky MA & Dorman DC (1994) Assessing risks of low-level methanol exposure. CIIT Act, **14**(7): 1-7.

Medinsky MA, Dorman DC, Bond JA, Moss OR, Janszen DB, & Everitt JI (1997) Pharmacokinetics of methanol and formate in female cynomolgus monkeys exposed to methanol vapours. Cambridge, Massachusetts, Health Effects Institute (Research Report No. 77).

Menne FR (1938) Acute methyl alcohol poisoning. Arch Pathol, **26**: 77-92.

Mill T, Hendry DG, & Richardson H (1980) Free-radical oxidants in natural waters. Science, **207**: 886-887.

Ministry of Supply and Services Canada (1993) Summary report 1993-A: National pollutant release inventory-Methanol air release. Ottawa, Ontario, Environment Canada, 11 pp.

Mohler FS & Gordon CJ (1990) Themoregulatory effects of methanol in Fischer and Long-Evans rats. Neurotoxicol Teratol, **12**: 41-45.

Mohr DH & King CJ (1985) Identification of polar organic compounds in coal-gasification condensate water by gas-chromatography-mass spectrometry analysis of high-performance liquid chromatography. Environ Sci Technol, **19**: 929-935.

Monte WC (1984) Aspartame: methanol and the public health. J Appl Nutr, **36**: 42-54.

Montgomery JH (1991) Groundwater chemicals desk reference. Chelsea, Michigan, Lewis Publishers, pp 491-495.

Morin AM & Liss M (1973) Evidence for a methylated protein intermediate in pituitary methanol formation. Biochem Biophys Res Commun, **52**: 373-378.

Morris GPL (1993) Renewed interest emerges for methanol, MTBE projects. Chem Week, **153**: 7.

Murray TG, Burton TC, Rajani C, Lewandowski MF, Burke JM, & Eells JT (1991) Methanol poisoning: A rodent model with structural and functional evidence for retinal involvement. Arch Ophthalmol, **109**: 1012-1016.

Naraqi S, Dethlefs RF, Slobodnuik RA, & Sairere JS (1979) An outbreak of acute methyl alcohol intoxication. Aust NZ J Med, **9**: 65-68.

National Poisons Information Service (1993) Antifreeze poisoning: Clinical effects and management. London, National Poisons Information Service, pp 1-4.

NEDO (1982) Toxicological research of methanol as a fuel for power station: Summary report on tests with monkeys, rats and mice. Tokyo, Japan, New Energy Development Organization.

NEDO (1987) Toxicological research of methanol as a fuel for power station: Summary report on tests with monkeys, rats and mice. Tokyo, Japan, New Energy Development Organization, pp 1-296.

Nelson BK, Brightwell WS, MacKenzie DR, Khan A, Burg JR, Weigel WW, & Goad PT (1985) Teratological assessment of methanol and ethanol at high inhalation levels in rats. Fundam Appl Toxicol, **5**: 727-736.

Nicholls P (1975) Formate as an inhibitor of cytochrome c oxidase. Biochem Biophys Res Commun, **67**: 610-616.

Nielsen IR, Malcolm HM, & Dobson SD (1993) Environmental hazard assessment: Methanol. Garston, Watford, UK Department of the Environment, Building Research Establishment, 45 pp.

NIOSH (1976) Criteria for a recommended standard .... Occupational exposure to methyl alcohol. Cincinnati, Ohio, National Institute for Occupational Safety and Health (HEW (NIOSH) Publication No. 76-148).

NIOSH (1977) NIOSH manual of analytical methods, 2nd ed. Cincinnati, Ohio, National Institute for Occupational Safety and Health (DHEW (NIOSH) Publication No. 77-157A).

NIOSH (1981) Health hazard evaluation report No. HETA-81-177, 178-988, University of Washington, Seattle. Cincinnati, Ohio, National Institute for Occupational Safety and Health.

NIOSH (1984) Method No. 2000: Methanol. In: Eller PM ed. NIOSH manual of analytical methods. Cincinnati, Ohio, National Institute for Occupational Safety and Health, vol 2, pp 2000/1-2000/4.

Noker PE, Eells JT, & Tephly TR (1980) Methanol toxicity: Treatment with folic acid and 5-formyl tetrahydrofolic acid alcoholism. Clin Exp Res, **4**: 378-383.

Norman V (1977) An overview of the vapor phase, semivolatile, and non-volatile components of cigarette smoke. Recent Adv Tob Sci, **3**: 25-58.

Novak JT, Goldsmith CD, Benoit RE, & O'Brien JH (1985) Biodegradation of methanol and tertiary butyl alcohol in subsurface systems. Water Sci Technol, **17**: 71-85.

Nyberg U, Aspegren H, Andersson B, Jansen JC, & Villadsen IS (1992) Full-scale application of nitrogen removal with methanol as carbon source. Water Sci Technol, **26**: 1077-1086.

Obe G & Ristow H (1977) Acetaldehyde, but not ethanol induces sister chromatid exchanges in Chinese hamster cells *in vitro*. Mutat Res, **56**: 211-213.

Okpokwasili GC & Amanchukwu SC (1988) Petroleum hydrocarbon degradation by candida species. Environ Int, **14**: 243-247.

Oliver B, Cosgrove EG, & Carey JH (1979) Effect of suspended sediments on the photolysis of organics in water. Environ Sci Technol, **13**: 1075-1077.

Ophaswongse S & Maibach HI (1994) Alcohol dermatitis: Allergic contact dermatitis and alcohol urtiaria syndrome. Contact Dermatitis, **30**: 1-6.

Oremland RS, Marsh LM, & Polcin S (1982) Methane production and simultaneous sulphite reduction in anoxic, salt marsh sediments. Nature (Lond), **296**: 143-145.

Owens LD, Gilbert RG, Griebel GE, & Menzies JD (1969) Identification of plant volatiles that stimulates microbial respiration and growth in soil. Phytopathology, **59**: 1468-1472.

Palese M & Tephly TE (1975) Metabolism of formate in the rat. J Toxicol Environ Health, **1**: 13-24.

Pamies RJ, Sugar D, Rives LA, & Herold AH (1993a) Methanol intoxication. Postgrad Med, **93**: 183-194.

Pamies RJ, Sugar D, Rives L, & Herold AH (1993b) Methanol intoxication: A case report. J Fla Med Assoc, **80**: 464-467.

Pankow S & Jagielki S (1993) Effect of methanol or modifications of the hepatic glutathione concentration on the metabolism of dichloromethane to carbon monoxide in rats. Hum Exp Toxicol, **12**: 227-231.

Pappas SC & Silverman M (1982) Treatment of methanol poisoning with ethanol and hemodialysis. Can Med Assoc J, **126**: 1391-1394.

Pappas AA, Gadsden RH, & Taylor EH (1985) Serum osmolality in acute intoxication: A prospective clinical study. Am J Clin Pathol, **84**: 74-79.

Pauls RE & McCoy RW (1981) Gas and liquid chromatographic analysis of methanol, ethanol, t-butanol and methyl-t-butyl ether in gasoline. J Chromatogr Sci, **19**: 558-561.

Pavlenko SM (1972) [Certain common traits in the action of industrial non-electrolyte poisons entering the body simultaneously with the water and air.] Gig I Sanit, **37**: 40-45 (in Russian).

Pearson A (1952) Acute methyl alcohol poisoning. Med J Aust, **2**: 437.

Pelletier J, Habib MH, Khalil R, Salamon G, Bartoli D, & Jean P (1992) Putaminal necrosis after methanol intoxication. J Neurol Neurosurg Psych, **55**: 234-235.

Pellizzari ED, Hartwell TD, Harris BSH III, Waddell RD, Whitaker DA, & Erikson MD (1982) Purgable organic compounds in mother's milk. Bull Environ Contam Toxicol, **28**: 322-328.

Pereira MA, Chang LW, McMillan L, Ward JB, & Legator MS (1982) Battery of short-term tests in laboratory animals to corroborate the detection of human population exposures to genotoxic chemicals. Environ Mutagen, **4**: 317.

Perkins RA, Ward KW, & Pollack GM (1995) A pharmacokinetic model of inhaled methanol in humans and comparison to methanol disposition in mice and rats. Environ Health Perspect, **103**: 716-733.

Phillips M & Greenberg J (1987) Detection of endogenous ethanol and other compounds in the breath by gas chromatography with on-column concentration of sample. Anal Biochem, **163**: 165-169.

Pienta RJ, Poiley JA, & Lebherz WB III (1977) Morphological transformation of early passage Golden Syrian hamster embryo cells derived from cryopreserved cultures as a reliable *in vitro* bioassay for identifying carcinogens. Int J Cancer, **19**: 642-655.

Pla A, Hernandez AF, Gil F, Garcia-Alonso M, & Villanueva E (1991) A fatal case of oral ingestion of methanol: Distribution in postmortem tissues and fluids including pericardial fluid and vitreous humor. Forensic Sci Int, **49**: 193-196.

Poirier SH, Knuth MI, Anderson-Buchou CD, Brooke CT, Lima AR, & Shubat PJ (1986) Comparative toxicity of methanol and N,N-dimethylformamide to freshwater fish and invertebrates. Bull Environ Contam Toxicol, **37**: 615-621.

Pollack GM & Brouwer KLR (1996) Maternal-fetal pharmacokinetics of methanol. Cambridge, Massachusetts, Health Effects Institute, 55 pp (Research Report No. 74).

Pollack GM & Kawagoe JL (1991) Determination of methanol in whole blood by capillary gas chromatography with direct on-column injection. J Chromatogr, **570**: 406-411.

Pollack GM, Brouwer KLR, & Kawagoe J (1993) Toxicokinetics of intravenous methanol in the female rat. Fundam Appl Toxicol, **21**: 105-110.

Poon R, Chu IH, Bjarnason S, Potvin M, Vincent R, Miller RB, & Valli VE (1994) Inhalation toxicity study of methanol, toluene and methanol/toluene mixtures in rats. Toxicol Ind Health, **10**: 231-245.

Poon R, Chu IH, Bjarnason S, Vincent R, Potvin M, Miller RB, & Valli VE (1995) Short-term inhalation toxicity of methanol, gasoline and methanol/gasoline in the rat. Toxicol Ind Health, **11**: 343-361.

Portmann JE & Wilson RW (1971) The toxicity of 140 substances to the brown shrimp and other marine animals. London, Ministry of Agriculture, Fisheries and Food (Shellfish Information Leaflet No. 22).

Posner HS (1975) Biohazards of methanol in proposed new uses. J Toxicol Environ Health, **1**: 153-171.

Price KS, Waggy GT, & Conway RA (1974) Brine shrimp bioassay and seawater BOD of petrochemicals. J Water Pollut Control Fed, **46**: 63-77.

Price EA, d'Alessandro A, Kearney T, Olson KR, & Blanc PD (1994) Osmolar gap with minimal acidosis in combined methanol and methyl ethyl ketone ingestion. Clin Toxicol, **32**: 79-84.

Rajini PS, Krishnakumari MK, & Majumder SK (1989) Cytotoxicity of certain organic solvents and organophosphorus insecticides to the ciliated protozoan *Paramecium caudatum*. Microbios, **59**: 157-163.

Rana SVS & Kumar S (1993a) Liver function in rats treated individually and with a combination of xylene, toluene and methanol. Toxicol Ind Health, **9**: 479-484.

Rana SVS & Kumar S (1993b) Effect of xylene, toluene and methyl alcohol on liver collagenesis in rats. Indian J Exp Biol, **31**: 782-784.

Randall TL & Knopp PV (1980) Detoxification of specific organic substances by wet oxidation. J Water Pollut Control Fed, **52**: 2117-2130.

Rastogi SC (1993) Organic solvents in model and hobby glues. Bull Environ Contam Toxicol, **51**: 501-507.

Reese E & Kimbrough RD (1994) Acute toxicity of gasoline and some additives. Environ Geochem Health, **101**(Suppl): 113-115.

Reisch MS (1994) Top 50 chemicals production rose modestly last year. Chem Eng News, **72**: 12-18.

Renzoni GE, Shankland EG, Gaines JA, & Callis JB (1985) Determination of alcohols in gasoline/alcohol blends by nuclear magnetic resonance spectrometry. Anal Chem, **57**: 2864-2867.

Rietbrock N (1969) [Kinetics and pathways of methanol metabolism.] Naunyn-Schmiedebergs Arch Pharmacol Exp Pathol, **263**: 189-201 (in German).

Rietbrock N, Stieren B, & Malorny G (1966) [Influence of folic acid on methanol metabolism.]. Klin Wochenschr, **44**: 1318.

Rippen G (1980) [Handbook of environmental chemicals.] Landsberg, Ecomed Verlagsgesellschaft, 16 pp (in German).

Röe O (1948) Methanol poisoning: The ganglion cells of the retina in cases of methanol poisoning in human beings and experimental animals. Acta Med Scand, **26**: 169-182.

Röe O (1950) The roles of alkaline salts and ethyl alcohol in the treatment of methanol poisoning. Q J Stud Alcohol, **11**: 107-112.

Röe O (1955) The metabolism and toxicity of methanol. Pharmacol Rev, **7**: 399-412.

Röe O (1982) Species differences in methanol poisoning. CRC Crit Rev Toxicol, **10**: 275-286.

Roeggla G, Wagner A, Frossard M, & Roeggla H (1993) Marked variability in methanol toxicity. Am Fam Physician, **48**: 731.

Rogers JM, Mole ML, Chernoff N, Barbee BD, Turner CI, Logsdon TR, & Kavlock RJ (1993) The developmental toxicity of inhaled methanol in the CD-1 mouse, with quantitative dose-response modeling for estimation of benchmark doses. Teratology, **47**: 175-188.

Rossini GDB & Ronco AE (1996) Acute toxicity bioassay using *Daphnia obtusa* as a test organism. Environ Toxicol Water Qual, **11**(3): 255-258.

Rotman D (1994a) Lurgi unveils route to methanol from carbon dioxide at ACS meeting. Chem Week, **154**: 14.

Rotman D (1994b) New approaches rekindle methanol conversion. Chem Week, **154**: 35.

Rowe VK & McCollister SB (1982) Alcohols. In: Clayton GD & Clayton FE ed. Parry's industrial hygiene and toxicology, 3rd ed. New York, John Wiley and Sons, vol 2C, pp 4528-4541.

Ruedemann AD (1962) The electroretinogram in chronic methyl alcohol poisoning in human beings. Am J Ophthalmol, **54**: 34-53.

Ryan BM, Hatoum NS, Mallett ES, & Yermakoff JK (1994) A pilot toxicity study of methanol in folate-deficient long-Evans rats. Teratology, **49**: 399.

Sakanashi TM, Rogers JM, & Keen CL (1994) Influence of folic acid intake on the developmental toxicity of methanol in the CD-1 mouse. Teratology, **49**: 368.

Sayers RR, Yant WP, & Schrenk HH (1942) Methanol poisoning exposure of dogs to 450-500 ppm methanol vapour in air. Washington, DC, US Bureau of Mines (Investigation Report No. 3619).

Sayers RR, Yant WP, Schrenk HH, Chornyak J, Pearce SJ, Patty FA, & Linn JG (1944) Methanol poisoning: II. Exposure of dogs for brief periods eight times daily to high concentrations of high methanol vapor in air. J Ind Hyg Toxicol, **26**: 255-259.

Scheunert I, Vockel D, Schnitzer J, & Korte F (1987) Bromineralization rates of ^{14}C-labelled organic chemicals in aerobic and anaerobic suspended soil. Chemosphere, **16**: 1031-1041.

Scheuplein RJ & Blank IH (1971) Permeability of the skin. Physiol Rev, **51**: 702-747.

Schiewe MH, Hawk EG, Actor DI, & Krahn MM (1985) Use of bacterial bioluminescence assay to access toxicity of contaminated marine sediments. Can J Fish Aquat Sci, **42**: 1244-1247.

Scholz B, Butzert H, Neumeister J, & Nierlich F (1990) Methyl tert-butyl ether. In: Elvers B, Hawkins S, Schutz G ed. Ullmann's encyclopedia of industrial chemistry, 5th ed. Weinheim, VCH Verlagsgesellschaft, vol 16a, pp 543-550.

Scott E, Helz MK, & McCord CP (1933) The histopathology of methyl alcohol poisoning. Am J Clin Pathol, **3**: 311-319.

Sedivec V, Mraz M, & Flek J (1981) Biological monitoring of persons exposed to methanol vapors. Int Arch Occup Environ Health, **48**: 257-271.

Seizinger DE & Dimitriades B (1972) Oxygenates in exhaust from simple hydrocarbon fuels. J Air Pollut Control Assoc, **22**: 47-51.

Sejersted OM, Jacobsen D, Ovrebo S, & Jansen H (1983) Formate concentration in plasma from patients poisoned with methanol. Acta Med Scand, **213**: 105-110.

Self R, Casey JC, & Swain T (1963) The low boiling volatiles of cooked foods. Chem Ind, **1963**: 863-864.

Sharpe JA, Hostovsky M, Bilbao JM, & Rewcastle NB (1982) Methanol optic neuropathy: A histopathological study. Neurology, **32**: 1093-1100.

Simmon VF, Kauhanen K, & Tardiff RG (1977) Mutagenic activity of chemicals identified in drinking water. In: Scott D, Bridges BA, & Sobels FH ed. Progress in genetic toxicology. Amsterdam, Elsevier/North Holland Press, vol 2, pp 249-268.

Simmons JE & McDonald A (1994) Effect of Kupffer cell inhibition on carbon tetrachloride hepatotoxicity in methanol pretreated rats. Toxicologist, **14**: 374.

Simmons JE, McDonald A, Seely JC & Sey YM (1995) ..... of carbon tetrachloride hepatotoxicity by inhaled methanol: Time course of recovery. J Toxicol Environ Health, **46**: 203-216.

Sims EW (1976) Determination of trace C_1-C_4 alcohols in aqueous solutions by gas chromatography. J Chromatogr Sci, **14**: 65-67.

Skaug OE (1956) A rapid and extremely sensitive test for methanol in blood and biological material. Scand J Clin Lab Invest, **8**: 338-339.

Smallwood AW (1978) Analysis of formic acid in air samples. Am Ind Hyg Assoc J, **39**: 151-153.

Smith NB (1984) Determination of volatile alcohols and acetone in serum by non-polar capillary gas chromatography after direct sample injection. Clin Chem, **30**: 1672-1674.

Smith EN & Taylor RT (1982) Acute toxicity of methanol in the folate-deficient acatalasemic mouse. Toxicology, **25**: 271-287.

Smyth HF, Seaton J, & Fischer L (1941) The single dose toxicity of some glycols and derivatives. J Ind Hyg Toxicol, **23**: 259-268.

Snider JR & Dawson GA (1985) Tropospheric light alcohols, carbonyls and acetonitrile: Concentrations in the Southwestern United States and Henry's law data. J Geophys Res, **90**: 3797-3805.

Snow R, Baker L, Crews W, Davis CO, Duncan J, Perry N, Siudak P, Stumpf K, Ray W, & Braddock J (1989) Characterization of emissions from a methanol fueled motor vehicle. J Air Pollut Control Assoc, **39**: 48-53.

SRI (1992) Chemical economics handbook: Marketing research report on methanol. Menlo Park, California, SRI International.

Stanton ME, Crofton KM, Gray LE, Gordon CM, Bushnell RJ, Mole ML, & Peale DB (1991) Assessment of offspring development and behavior following gestational exposure to inhaled methanol in the rat. Toxicologist, **11**: 118.

Stanton ME, Crofton KM, Gray LE, Gordon CJ, Boyes WK, Mole ML, Peele DB, & Bushnell PS (1995) Assessment of offspring development and behaviour following gestational exposure to inhaled methanol in the rat. Fundam Appl Toxicol, **28**: 100-110.

Stegink LD, Brummel MC, McMartin KE, Martin-Amat G, Filer LJ Jr, Baker GL, & Tephly TR (1981) Blood methanol concentrations in normal adult subjects administered abuse doses of aspartame. J Toxicol Environ Health, **7**: 281-290.

Stegink LD, Brummel MC, Filer LJ Jr, & Baker GL (1983) Blood methanol concentrations in one-year-old infants administered graded doses of aspartame. J Nutr, **113**: 1600-1606.

Stensel HD, Loehr RC, & Lawrence AW (1973) Biological kinetics of suspended-growth denitrification. J Water Pollut Control Fed, **45**: 249-261.

Stern S, Reuhl K, Soderholm S, Cox C, Sharma A, Balys M, Gelein R, Yin C, & Weiss B (1996) Perinatal methanol exposure in the rat: I. Blood methanol concentration and neural cell adhesion molecules. Fundam Appl Toxicol, **34**: 36-46.

Stratton GW (1985) The influence of solvent type on solvent-pesticide interactions in bioassays. Arch Environ Contam Toxicol, **14**: 651-658.

Stratton GW (1987) Toxic effects of organic solvents on the growth of blue-green algae. Bull Environ Contam Toxicol, **38**: 1012-1019.

Stratton GW & Smith TM (1988) Interaction of organic solvents with the green alga *Chlorella pyrenoidosa*. Bull Environ Contam Toxicol, **40**: 736-742.

Strittmatter P & Ball EG (1955) Formaldehyde dehydrogenase, a glutathione-dependent enzyme system. J Biol Chem, **213**: 445.

Suit PF & Estes M (1990) Methanol intoxication: clinical features and differential diagnosis. Clevel Clin J Med, **57**: 464-471.

Swain HM & Somerville HJ (1978) Microbial metabolism of methanol in a model activated sludge system. J Appl Bacteriol, **45**: 147-151.

Swartz RD, Millman RP, Billi JE, Bondar NP, Migdal SD, Simonian SK, Monforte JR, McDonald FD, Harness JK, & Cole KL (1981) Epidemic methanol poisoning: clinical and biochemical analysis of a recent episode. Medicine, **60**: 373-382.

Sweger DM & Travis JC (1979) An application of infrared lasers to the selective detection of trace organic gases. Appl Spectrom, **33**: 46-51.

Tackett SI (1987) Determination of methanol in gasoline by gas chromatography. Analyst, **112**: 339-340.

Takagi H, Hatakeyama S, Akimoto H, & Koda S (1986) Formation of methyl nitrite in the surface reaction of nitrogen dioxide and methanol: 1. Dark reaction. Environ Sci Technol, **20**: 387-393.

Tephly TR (1991) Mini review-the toxicity of methanol. Life Sci, **48**: 1031-1041.

Tephly TR & McMartin KE (1984) Methanol metabolism and toxicity. In: SteginK LD & Filer LJ Jr ed. Aspartame: Physiology and biochemistry. New York, Basel, Marcel Dekker, pp 111-140.

Tephly TR, Parks RE, & Mannering GJ (1964) Methanol metabolism in the rat. J Pharmacol Exp Ther, **143**: 292-300.

Teschke R, Masamura Y, & Lieber CS (1975) Hepatic microsomal alcohol-oxidising system: affinity for methanol, ethanol, propanol and butanol. J Biol Che,. **250**: 7397.

Tichy M, Trcka V, Roth Z, & Krivucova M (1985) QSAR analysis and data extrapolation among mammals in a series of aliphatic alcohols. Environ Health Perspect, **61**: 321-328.

Tonning DJ, Brooks DW, & Harlow CM (1956) Acute methyl alcohol poisonings in 49 naval ratings. Can Med Assoc J, **74**: 20-27.

Triebig G & Schaller KH (1980) A simple and reliable enzymatic assay for the determination of formic acid in urine. Clin Chim Acta, **108**: 355-360

Tyson HH & Schoenberg MJ (1914) Experimental researches in methyl alcohol inhalation. J Am Med Assoc, **63**: 915-921.

Ubaidullaev R (1966) [Effect of small concentrations of methanol vapours on the body of men and animals.] Gig I Sanit, **31**: 9-12 (in Russian).

UK Standing Committee of Analysts (1982) Formaldehyde, methanol and related compounds in raw, waste and potable waters: Methods for the examination of waters and associated materials, London, UK Standing Committee of Analysts, Her Majesty Stationery Office.

Uotila L & Koivusalo M (1974) Formaldehyde dehydrogenase from human liver: Purification, properties and evidence for the formation of glutathione thiol esters by the enzyme. J Biol Chem, **249**: 7653.

Upadhyay S & Gupta VK (1984) Reagent system for the spectrophotometric determination of methanol in environmental and biological samples. Analyst, **109**: 1427-1429.

Upton J (1993) Denitrification of sewage effluents in deep bed sand filters. Water Sci Technol, **27**: 381-390.

US EPA (1975) Identification of organic compounds in effluents from industrial sources. Washington, DC, US Environmental Protection Agency, Office of Toxic Substances (EPA 560-3-75-002).

US EPA (1976a) Assessment of methyl alcohol as a potential air pollution problem - Volume II. Research Triangle Park, North Carolina, US Environmental Protection Agency (NTIS Publication No. PB-258354).

US EPA (1976b) Frequency of organic compounds identified in water. Washington, DC, US Environmental Protection Agency (EPA 600/4-76-062).

US EPA (1977) Multimedia environmental goals for environmental assessment - Volume II: MEG, charts and background information. Washington, DC, US Environmental Protection Agency, pp E28-E29 (EPA 600/7-77-126b).

US EPA (1979) Atmospheric reaction products of organic compounds. Washington, DC, US Environmental Protection Agency, 80 pp (Report No. PB 301-384, prepared by SRI International, Menlo Park, California).

US EPA (1980a) Chemical hazard information profiles (CHIPS). Washington, DC, US Environmental Protection Agency (EPA 560/11-80-011).

US EPA (1980b) Organic chemical manufacturing - Volume 9: Selected processes. Research Triangle Park, North Carolina, US Environmental Protection Agency (EPA 450/3-80-028d).

US EPA (1983) Toxicity and metabolism studies with EPA priority pollutants and related chemicals in freshwater organisms. Washington, DC, US Environmental Protection Agency.

US EPA (1988) Toxic air pollutant emission factors: A compilation for selected air toxic compounds and sources. Research Triangle Park, North Carolina, US Environmental Protection Agency (EPA 450/2-88-006).

US EPA (1991) Urban formaldehyde and methanol concentrations for alternative methanol vehicle scenarios. Research Triangle Park, North Carolina, US Environmental Protection Agency (Report No. CRC-APRAC-ME-2).

US EPA (1993) Ambient concentration summaries for Clean Air Act, Title III: Hazardous air pollutants. Washington, DC, US Environmental Protection Agency, p B-17 (EPA 600/R-94-090).

US EPA (1994) 1992 Toxic release inventory: Public data. Washington, DC, US Environmental Protection Agency (EPA 745/R-94-001).

US NIOSH (1976) Recommended standard for occupational exposure to methyl alcohol. Cincinnati, Ohio, National Institute for Occupational Safety and Health, 136 pp.

Vaishnav DD & Korthals ET (1990) Comparative toxicities of selected industrial chemicals to microorganisms and other aquatic organisms. Arch Environ Contam Toxicol, **19**: 624-628.

Vaishnav DD & Lopas DM (1985) Relationship between lipophilicity and biodegradation inhibition of selected industrial chemicals. Dev Ind Microbiol, **26**: 557-565.

Veith GD, Call DJ, & Brooke LT (1983) Structure-toxicity relationships for the fat-head minnow, *Pimephales promelas*: narcotic industrial chemicals. Can J Fish Aquat Sci, **40**: 743-748.

Vendilo MV, Egorov YL, & Feldman NG (1971) [The effects of methanol and of some higher alcohols on the retina of the eyes (an electron-microscope investigation).] Gig Tr Prof Zabol, **15**: 17-21 (in Russian).

Venkataraman ES, Ahlert RC, & Corbo P (1984) Biological treatment of landfill leachates. CRC Crit Rev Environ Control, **14**: 333-376.

Verma P & Gupta VK (1984) A sensitive spectrophotometric method for the determination of methyl alcohol in air and water. Talanta, **31**: 394-396.

Vogt MJ, Heffner JE, & Sahn SA (1993) Vomiting, abdominal pain and visual disturbances in a 31-year old man. Chest, **103**: 262-263.

Ward KW & Pollack GM (1996a) Comparative toxicokinetics of methanol in pregnant and nonpregnant rodents. Drug Metab Dispos, **24**: 1062-1070.

Ward KW & Pollack GM (1996b) Use of intrauterine microdialysis to investigate methanol-induced alterations in uteroplacental blood flow. Toxicol Appl Pharmacol, **140**: 203-210.

Ward JB, Hokanson JA, Smith ER, Chang LW, Pereira MA, Whorton EB, & Legator MS (1984) Sperm count, morphology and fluorescent body frequency in autopsy workers exposed to formaldehyde. Mutat Res, **130**: 417-424.

Ward KW, Perkins RA, Kawagoe JL, & Pollack GM (1995) Comparative toxicokinetics of methanol in the female mouse and rat. Fundam Appl Toxicol, **26**: 258-264.

Weese H (1928) Vergleichende untersuchungen uber die wirksamkeit und giftigkeit der dampfe niederer aliphatischer alkohole. Arch Exptl Pathol Pharmacol, 135: 118-130 [in German].

Weiss B, Stern S, Soderholm SC, Cox C, Sharma A, Inglis GB, Preston R, Balys M, Reuhl KR, & Gelein R (1996) Developmental neurotoxicity of methanol exposure by inhalation in rats. Cambridge, Massachusetts, Health Effects Institute (Research Report No. 73).

Welch H & Slocum GG (1943) Toxicity of methanol. J Lab Chem Med, **28**: 1440-1445.

Wenzyl JE, Mills SD, & McCall JT (1968) Methanol poisoning in an infant. Am J Dis Child, **116**: 445-447.

Whitbeck M (1983) Photo-oxidation of methanol. Atmos Environ, **17**: 121-126.

White LR, Martinsen ABL, & Nilsen OG (1983) Biochemical and cytological studies of rat lung after inhalation of methanol vapour. Toxicol Lett, **17**: 1-5.

WHO (1971) Evaluation of food additives. Fourteenth report of the Joint FAO/WHO Expert Committee on Food Additives. Geneva, World Health Organization, p 20 (WHO Technical Report Series No. 462).

Williams RL, Lipari F, & Potter RA (1990) Formaldehyde, methanol and hydrocarbon emissions from methanol-fueled cars. J Air Waste Manage Assoc, **40**: 747-756.

Windholz M ed. (1983) The Merck index: An encyclopedia of chemicals, drugs and biologicals, 10th ed. Rahway, New Jersey, Merck & Co.,Inc., p 853.

Wood CA & Buller F (1904) Poisoning by wood alcohol. J Am Med Assoc, **43**: 973-977.

Wu Chen NB, Donoghue ER, & Schaffer MI (1985) Methanol intoxication: Distribution in postmortem tissues and fluids including vitreous humor. J Forensic Sci, **30**: 213-216.

Wucherpfennig K, Dietrich H, & Bechtel J (1983) Alcohol actual, total and potential methyl alcohol of fruit juices. Flussiges Obst, **8**: 348-354.

Yant WP & Schrenk HH (1937) Distribution of methanol in dogs after inhalation and administration by stomach tube and subcutaneously. J Ind Hyg Toxicol, **19**: 337-345.

Yasugi T, Kawai T, Mizunuma K, Horiguchi S, Iwami O, Iguchi H, & Ikeda M (1992) Formic acid excretion in comparison with methanol excretion in urine of workers occupationally exposed to methanol. Int Arch Occup Environ Health, **64**: 329-337.

Youssef AF, Baggs RB, Weiss B, & Miller RK (1991) Methanol teratogenicity in pregnant Long-Evans rats. Teratology, **43**: 467.

Youssef AF, Madkour K, Cox C, & Weiss B (1992) Comparative lethality of methanol, ethanol and mixtures in female rats. J Appl Toxicol, **12**: 193-197.

Youssef AF, Weiss B, & Cox C (1993) Neurobehavioural toxicity of methanol reflected by operant running. Neurotoxicol Teratol, **15**: 223-227.

Zinbo M (1984) Determination of one-carbon to three-carbon alcohols and water in gasoline/alcohol blends by liquid chromatography. Anal Chem, **56**: 244-247.

RESUME

1.   Identité, propriétés physiques et chimiques et méthodes d'analyse

Le méthanol se présente sous la forme d'un liquide incolore et limpide qui dégage une légère odeur alcoolique à l'état pur. Volatil et inflammable, il est miscible à l'eau et à de nombreux solvants organiques et forme un grand nombre d'azéotropes binaires.

Il existe un certain nombre de méthodes, principalement la chromatographie en phase gazeuse avec détection par ionisation de flamme, pour la recherche et le dosage du méthanol dans divers échantillons prélevés dans l'environnement (air, eau, sol, et sédiments) ou dans les produits alimentaires. Ces méthodes sont également utilisées pour la recherche et le dosage du méthanol et de son principal métabolite, le formiate, dans les liquides et les tissus biologiques. Outre la chromatographie en phase gazeuse ave détection par ionisation de flamme, il existe des méthodes enzymatiques colorimétriques pour le dosage du formiate dans le sang, les urines et les tissus.

Pour les analyses sur le lieu de travail, on commence généralement par recueillir et concentrer l'échantillon sur gel de silice, après quoi on procède à une extraction par l'eau, puis au dosage proprement dit par chromatographie en phase gazeuse avec détection par ionisation de flamme ou spectrométrie de masse.

2.   Sources d'exposition humaine

Le méthanol est présent à l'état naturel chez l'Homme, les animaux et les plantes. C'est un constituant du sang, de l'urine, de la salive et de l'air expiré. On a mesuré des concentrations moyennes de méthanol égales à 0,73 mg/litre dans les urines (valeurs extrêmes:0,3-2,61 mg/litre) chez des sujets non exposés et des valeurs allant de 0,06 à 0,32 µg/litre ont été observées dans l'air expiré.

Le méthanol et le formiate naturellement présents dans l'organisme proviennent essentiellement de deux sources: l'alimentation et le métabolisme. Le méthanol d'origine alimentaire est principalement apporté par les fruits et les légumes frais ainsi que par les jus de fruits (teneur moyenne: 140 mg/litre avec des valeurs extrêmes de 12-640 mg/litre), les boissons fermentées (jusqu'à 1,5 g/litre), et autres composants du régime alimentaire (principalement les boissons non alcoolisées). L'aspartame est un édulcorant très utilisé dont l'hydrolyse donne du méthanol absorbable dans la proportion de 10% en poids.

En 1991, la production mondiale de méthanol a atteint environ 20 millions de tonnes, principalement par conversion catalytique de gaz de synthèse sous pression (hydrogène, dioxyde et monoxyde de carbone). La capacité mondiale de production devrait atteindre 30 millions de tonnes en 1995.

Le méthanol est utilisé dans l'industrie pour la production de nombreux produits chimiques importants, principalement le méthyltertiobutyléther, le formaldéhyde, l'acide acétique, les éthers méthyliques du glycol, la méthylamine, les halogénures de méthyle et le méthacrylate de méthyle.

Le méthanol entre dans la composition de nombreux solvants du commerce et de divers produits comme les peintures, les laques, les vernis, les diluants pour peintures, les détachants, les antigels, les liquides pour pare-brise, les dégivrants, les produits pour la photocopie, les solutions destinées à la dénaturation de l'éthanol ainsi que différent types de colles. Le méthanol pourrait également être utilisé directement comme combustible, ou bien encore être ajouté à l'essence à titre de combustible auxiliaire ou de diluant. Il est à noter que les cas les plus fréquents d'intoxication, mortelle ou non, par le méthanol, sont dus à l'ingestion volontaire ou accidentelle de produits qui en contiennent.

On a trouvé du méthanol dans les gaz d'échappement des moteurs à essence et des moteurs diesel ainsi que dans la fumée de tabac.

3. Concentrations dans l'environnement et exposition humaine

Les émissions de méthanol proviennent essentiellement des divers usages qui en sont faits en tant que solvant industriel ou domestique, des unités de production du composé lui-même ou de ses dérivés, enfin des pertes lors du stockage ou de la manipulation.

Il peut y avoir exposition au méthanol sur le lieu de travail par inhalation ou contact cutané. A en juger d'après les limites d'exposition fixées par de nombreux pays, il semblerait que les travailleurs ne courent pas de danger tant que l'exposition exprimée en moyenne pondérée par rapport au temps ne dépasse pas 260 mg/m^3 (200 ppm) par journée de 8 h et semaine de 40 h.

Actuellement la population est exposée à des concentrations qui sont 10 000 fois inférieures aux limites d'exposition professionnelle. En ce qui concerne l'exposition au méthanol contenu dans l'air, les concentrations vont de 0,001 mg/m^3 (0,8 parties par milliard) en milieu rural, à près de 0,04 mg/m^3 (30 parties par milliard) en milieu urbain.

On ne possède guère de données sur la teneur en méthanol de l'eau de boisson après traitement, mais ce composé est en tout cas souvent présent dans les effluents industriels.

Si les prévisions d'utilisation du méthanol comme combustible de substitution ou d'appoint augmentent de façon sensible, il faut s'attendre à ce que l'exposition à ce composé se généralise par suite de l'inhalation des vapeurs émises par les véhicules qui l'utiliseront,ou encore de son siphonage ou de son absorption percutanée lors de la manipulation de combustibles qui en contiendront.

4. Distribution et transformation dans l'environnement

Le méthanol se décompose rapidement dans l'environnement par photooxydation et sous l'action de processus de biodégration. Dans le cas de la réaction atmosphérique du méthanol avec les radicaux hydroxyle, on a mesuré une demi-vie de 7 à 18 jours.

De nombreux genres et souches de microorganismes sont capables d'utiliser le méthanol comme substrat. Le composé est facilement dégradé en aérobiose ou en anaérobiose dans des milieux très divers, notamment les eaux douces ou salées, les sols et les sédiments, les eaux souterraines, les nappes phréatiques et les effluents industriels. En général, 70% du méthanol présent dans les eaux d'égout est décomposé en l'espace de 5 jours.

Le méthanol sert normalement de substrat à de nombreux microorganismes terricoles, qui sont capables de le dégrader complètement en dioxyde carbone et en eau.

Le méthanol est médiocrement absorbé par les sols. Sa bioaccumulation est faible dans la plupart des organismes.

Le méthanol est peu toxique pour les organismes aquatiques et terrestres et il est peu probable que l'on observe des effets résultant d'une exposition environnementale à ce composé, sauf en cas de déversements dans la nature.

5. Absorption, distribution, biotransformation et élimination

Après inhalation, ingestion ou contact cutané, le méthanol est facilement résorbé et se diffuse rapidement dans les tissus en fonction de la répartition de l'eau dans l'organisme. Une faible proportion est excrétée telle quelle par les poumons et les reins.

Après ingestion, les concentrations sériques maximales sont atteintes en 30 à 90 minutes et le méthanol se répartit dans l'organisme avec un volume de distribution d'environ 0,6 litre/kg.

Le méthanol est métabolisé principalement au niveau du foie selon un processus oxydatif qui le transforme successivement en formaldéhyde, acide formique et dioxyde de carbone. La première étape, celle de l'oxydation en formaldéhyde, s'effectue sous l'action de l'alcool-déshydrogénase hépatique; il s'agit d'une étape limitante qui correspond à un processus saturable. L'affinité relative de l'alcool-déshydrogénase pour le méthanol et pour l'éthanol est d'environ 20:1. Lors de la seconde étape, le formaldéhyde est oxydé par la formaldéhyde - déshydrogénase en acide formique ou en formiate, selon la valeur du pH. La troisième étape consiste dans la détoxication de l'acide formique en dioxyde de carbone par des réactions dépendant de l'acide folique.

L'élimination du méthanol présent dans le sang par la voie urinaire ou dans l'air expiré, soit tel quel, soit après métabolisation, se révèle être un processus lent chez toutes les espèces, en particulier par comparaison avec l'éthanol. Ainsi, la clairance du méthanol s'effectue avec une demi-vie de 24 h ou davantage pour des doses inférieures à 0,1 g/kg. C'est au niveau de la détoxication métabolique, c'est-à-dire de l'élimination du formiate, que des différences très importantes existent entre les rongeurs et les primates et ce sont elles qui expliquent la différence spectaculaire de toxicité que l'on constate entre les premiers et les seconds.

6. Effets sur les mammifères de laboratoire et les systèmes d'épreuve *in vitro*

6.1 *Toxicité générale*

La toxicité aiguë et la toxicité à court terme du méthanol varient beaucoup selon les diverses espèces et elles sont maximales chez celles qui métabolisent relativement mal le formiate. En pareil cas, le méthanol provoque une intoxication mortelle par acidose métabolique et toxicité neuronale. En revanche, chez les animaux qui métabolisent bien le formiate, la mort survient habituellement par suite de la dépression du système nerveux central (coma, insuffisance respiratoire etc.). Chez les primates sensibles (comme l'Homme et les singes), il y a augmentation du taux sanguin de formiate après exposition au méthanol, alors que chez les rongeurs résistants, les lapins et les chiens, cette augmentation du taux de formiate ne se produit pas. L'Homme et les primates non humains présentent une sensibilité unique aux effets toxiques du méthanol. Globalement, le méthanol est peu toxique pour les animaux autres que les primates. La valeur de la DL_{50} et de la dose létale minimale pour une exposition par la voie orale, varie de 7000 à 13 000 mg/kg chez le rat, la souris, le lapin et le chien et de 2000 à 7000 mg/kg chez le singe.

Chez des rats exposés à du méthanol 6 h par jour, 5 jours par semaine pendant 4 semaines, à des concentrations allant jusqu'à 6500 mg/m^3 (5000 ppm), on n'a observé aucun effet imputable à l'exposition, sauf une augmentation des écoulements au niveau du nez et des yeux. On estime qu'il s'agissait là de la conséquence d'une irritation des voies respiratoires supérieures.

Des rats exposés à des vapeurs de méthanol à des concentrations pouvant atteindre 13 000 mg/m^3 (10 000 ppm), 6 h par jour, 5 jours par semaine pendant 6 semaines, n'ont pas présenté de signes de toxicité pulmonaire.

Chez le lapin, le méthanol irrite modérément la muqueuse oculaire. Lors d'une épreuve qui était une variante du test de maximalisation, il n'a pas provoqué de sensibilisation cutanée.

Parmi les effets toxiques du méthanol observés chez les primates, on peut citer l'acidose métabolique et la toxicité oculaire qui ne se produisent en principe pas chez les rongeurs dont le taux de folate est suffisant. Ces différences de toxicité s'expliquent par des différences dans la vitesse de métabolisation du formiate, qui est un métabolite du méthanol. Par exemple, la clairance du formiate sanguin est au moins 50% plus lente chez les primates que chez les rongeurs.

Des singes qui recevaient du méthanol par gavage à des doses dépassant 3000 mg/kg ont présenté une ataxie, de la faiblesse et une léthargie dans les quelques heures suivant l'administration du composé. Ces signes avaient tendance à disparaître en l'espace de 24 h et ils étaient suivis d'un coma passager chez certains des animaux.

Chez des singes exposés à du méthanol à 20 reprises 6 h par jour et 5 jours par semaines, à la dose de 6500 mg/m^3 (5000 ppm), on n'a pas constaté d'effets oculaires.

6.2 Génotoxicité et cancérogénicité

Les tests de mutation génétique effectués avec du méthanol sur des bactéries et des levures ont donné des résultats négatifs, mais le composé à provoqué une ségrégation chromosomique défectueuse chez *Aspergillus*. Il n'a pas provoqué d'échanges de chromatides soeurs dans des cellules de hamster chinois *in vitro*, mais il a augmenté de façon sensible la fréquence des mutations dans des cellules lymphomateuses de souris L5178Y.

L'inhalation de méthanol n'a pas provoqué de lésions chromosomiques chez la souris. Par contre, on est fondé à penser, dans une certaine mesure, que l'administration intrapéritonéale ou buccale de méthanol augmente l'incidence des lésions chromosomiques chez la souris.

Rien n'indique, au vu de l'expérimentation animale, que le méthanol soit cancérogène, mais il faut admettre qu'il n'existe pas de modèle animal approprié pour ce genre d'étude.

6.3 *Toxicité pour la fonction reproductrice, embryotoxicité et tératogénicité*

Des études concernant les effets sur les taux de gonadotrophine et de testostérone d'une exposition au méthanol, par la voie respiratoire, pendant des périodes allant jusqu'à 6 semaines, ont donné des résultats contradictoires.

En faisant inhaler du méthanol à des rongeurs gravides pendant toute la période de l'embryogénèse, on obtient toute une série d'effets tératogènes et embryocides qui dépendent de la concentration. Ainsi, on a observé des malformations attribuables au traitement et consistant principalement dans la présence de côtes cervicales surnuméraires ou rudimentaires, ou encore de malformations urinaires ou cardio-vasculaires, chez des foetus de rats exposés 7 h par jour du 7iéme au 15 ième jour de la gestation à une concentration de 26 000 mg/m^3, soit l'équivalent de 20 000 ppm, de méthanol. A cette concentration, le méthanol était légèrement toxique pour les mères. En revanche, à la concentration de 6500 mg/m^3 (5000 ppm), aucun effet indésirable n'a été noté chez les mères ou chez leur progéniture et on a considéré que cette valeur constituait la concentration sans effet nocif observable (NOAEL) pour ce système d'épreuve.

Dans la progéniture de souris CD-1 exposées à du méthanol à des concentrations supérieures ou égales à 6500 mg/m^3 (5000 ppm), 7 h par jour du 6 ième au 15 ième jour de la gestation, on a observé une incidence accrue d'exencéphalies et de fissures de la voûte palatine. Aux concentrations supérieures ou égales à 9825 mg/m^3 (7500 ppm), les résorptions affectant la totalité de la portée étaient également plus fréquentes. Aux concentrations de 13 000 et 19 500 mg/m^3 (10 000 ou 15 000 ppm), on a observé une réduction du poids foetal. La concentration sans effet observable (NOAEL) sur le développement a été évaluée à 1300 mg/m^3 (1000 ppm). Aux concentrations inférieures à 9000 mg/m^3 (7000 ppm), rien n'a été relevé qui puisse indiquer une toxicité du méthanol pour les mères.

En donnant à la progéniture de ces souris CD-1 une dose de 4 g/kg de méthanol par gavage, on a constaté que l'incidence des effets nocifs (résorptions, fissures palatines et réduction du poids foetal) était analogue à celle constatée dans le groupe de rats auxquels on avait fait inhaler le composé à la concentration de 13 000 mg/m^3 (10 000 ppm), probablement en raison de la fréquence respiratoire plus élevée chez la souris. La souris est plus sensible que le rat aux effets toxiques que le méthanol inhalé exerce sur le développement.

Des signes neurologiques passagers et une réduction du poids corporel ont été enregistrés chez des souris CD-1 gravides, exposées 6 h par jour à une concentration de 19 500 mg/m^3, soit l'équivalent de 15 000 ppm tout au long de l'organogénèse (du sixième au quinzième jour). Parmi les malformations foetales observées aux doses de 19 500 et 13 000 mg/m^3, soit 15 000 et 10 000 ppm, on peut citer des anomalies neurales et oculaires, des fissures palatines, des hydronéphroses et des malformations des membres.

7. Effets sur l'Homme

L'Homme (et les primates non humains) présentent une sensibilité unique au méthanol et les effets toxiques relevés chez ces espèces sont caractérisés par une acidémie formique, une acidose métabolique, une toxicité oculaire, une dépression du système nerveux, la cécité, le coma et la mort. Presque toutes les données que l'on possède sur la toxicité du méthanol pour l'Homme, ont trait aux conséquences des intoxications aiguës plutôt qu'à celles des intoxications chroniques. La très grande majorité des intoxications par le méthanol résultent de la consommation de boissons frelatées et de produits contenant du méthanol. C'est par ingestion que se produisent la plupart de ces intoxications, mais l'inhalation de vapeurs de méthanol sous forte concentration et l'absorption percutanée de solutions méthanoliques conduisent aux mêmes effets toxiques que l'ingestion. Les effets toxiques les plus fréquemment notés à la suite d'une exposition de longue durée, sont des effets oculaires très variés.

Les effets toxiques du méthanol sont liés aux facteurs qui régissent la conversion du méthanol en acide formique et la transformation ultérieure de ce dernier en dioxyde de carbone par la voie des folates. Ces effets se manifestent lorsque la vitesse de formation du formiate est supérieure à sa vitesse de métabolisation.

On ne sait pas avec certitude quelle est la dose mortelle pour l'Homme. En l'absence d'intervention médicale, la dose létale minimum se situe entre 0,3 et 1 g/kg. On ignore quelle est dose minimale à partir de laquelle se produisent des lésions oculaires permanentes.

L'acidose métabolique est de gravité variable et elle n'est pas forcément en bonne corrélation avec la quantité de méthanol ingérée. Les intoxications méthanoliques se caractérisent par de grandes variations individuelles dans la dose toxique.

Il semble que deux facteurs importants déterminent la sensibilité humaine aux effets toxiques du méthanol: 1) l'ingestion simultanée d'éthanol, qui retarde l'entrée du méthanol dans sa voie de dégradation métabolique; 2) le bilan des folates hépatiques, dont dépend la vitesse de détoxication du formiate.

Les symptômes de l'intoxication méthanolique, qui peuvent ne se manifester qu'au bout de 12 à 24 h, consistent en troubles visuels, nausées, douleurs abdominales et musculaires, étourdissements, faiblesse et troubles de la conscience allant du coma au crises cloniques. Les troubles visuels apparaissent généralement dans les 12 à 18 h suivant l'ingestion de méthanol et vont d'une légère photophobie avec une vision floue ou voilée à une réduction importante de l'acuité visuelle, voire à la cécité totale. Dans les cas extrêmes, l'intoxication peut avoir une issue fatale. Sur le plan clinique, la principale manifestation est une acidose métabolique grave par augmentation du trou anionique. L'acidose est largement attribuée à l'acide formique résultant de la métabolisation du méthanol.

La concentration sanguine normale du méthanol d'origine endogène est inférieure à 0,5 mg/litre (0,02 mmol/litre), mais l'alimentation peut accroître le taux sanguin de méthanol. En général, les effets neurologiques centraux apparaissent lorsque la concentration sanguine du méthanol dépasse 200 mg/litre (6 mmol/litre); les symptômes oculaires se manifestent à partir de 500 mg/litre (16 mmol/litre) et la mort est survenue chez des patients non traités dont les taux sanguins initiaux de méthanol se situaient entre 1500 et 2000 mg/litre, soit 47 à 62 mmol/litre.

L'inhalation occasionnelle de vapeurs de méthanol à une concentration inférieure à 260 mg/m^3 ou l'ingestion du liquide en quantités ne dépassant pas 20 mg/kg, ne devraient pas conduire à une accumulation de formiate supérieure au taux endogène, s'agissant de sujets en bonne santé ou présentant un déficit modéré en folate. Des troubles visuels de divers types (vision floue, rétrécissement du champ visuel, modification de la perception des couleurs et cécité temporaire ou permanente) ont été signalés chez des travailleurs exposés à des concentrations de méthanol dans l'air inférieures ou égales à environ 1500 mg/m^3 (1200 ppm).

On utilise largement la valeur de 260 mg/m^3 (200 ppm) comme limite d'exposition professionnelle au méthanol. Cette valeur a été calculée pour protéger les travailleurs contre l'acidose formique induite par le méthanol et contre les effets toxiques de ce composé sur l'oeil et le système nerveux.

On n'a pas signalé chez l'Homme d'autres effets nocifs qu'une légère irritation cutanée et oculaire aux concentrations très supérieures à 260 mg/m^3 (200 ppm).

8. Effets sur les êtres vivants dans leur milieu naturel

Pour les organismes aquatiques, la valeur de la CL_{50} varie de 1300 à 15 900 mg/litre dans le cas des invertébrés (exposition de 48 h et de 96 h), et de 13 000 à 29 000 mg/litre dans le cas des poissons (exposition de 96 h).

Le méthanol est peu toxique pour les organismes aquatiques et il n'est guère probable que l'on observe des effets imputables à une exposition environnementale, sauf en cas de déversement de méthanol dans la nature.

RESUMEN

1. Identidad propiedades físicas y químicas y métodos analíticos

El metanol es un líquido transparente, incoloro, volátil e inflamable con un ligero olor alcohólico en estado puro. Se puede mezclar con el agua y con muchos disolventes orgánicos y forma numerosas mezclas azeotrópicas binarias.

Hay métodos analíticos, principalmente la cromatografía de gases (CG) con detección por ionización de llama (DIL), para la determinación del metanol en diversos medios (aire, agua, suelo y sedimentos) y productos alimenticios, así como para la determinación del metanol y de su principal metabolito, el formiato, en los líquidos y tejidos corporales. Además de la CG-DIL, en la determinación del formiato en la sangre, la orina y los tejidos se utilizan procedimientos enzimáticos con resultados finales colorimétricos.

Para la determinación del metanol en el lugar de trabajo se suele comenzar con la recolección y concentración en silicagel, seguida de extracción acuosa y CG-DIL o análisis de CG-espectrometría de masa del extracto.

2. Fuentes de exposición humana

El metanol está presente de forma natural en el ser humano, los animales y las plantas. Es un elemento constitutivo natural en la sangre, orina, la saliva y el aire expirado. Se ha descrito una concentración media de metanol en orina de 0,73 mg/litro (intervalo de 0,3-2,61 µg/litro) en individuos no expuestos y una gama de 0,06 a 0,32 µg/litro en el aire expirado.

Las dos fuentes más importantes de acumulación básica de metanol y formiato en el organismo son la alimentación y los procesos metabólicos. El metanol está disponible en la alimentación principalmente a partir de las frutas y hortalizas frescas, los zumos de fruta (promedio de 140 mg/litro, margen de variación de 12 a 640 mg/litro), las bebidas fermentadas (hasta 1,5 g/litro) y los alimentos de dieta (sobre todo bebidas no alcohólicas). El aspartame es un edulcorante artificial muy utilizado, y al hidrolizarse el 10% (por peso) de la molécula se convierte en metanol libre, que queda disponible para la absorción.

En 1991 se produjeron en todo el mundo alrededor de 20 millones de toneladas de metanol, fundamentalmente por conversión catalítica de gas de síntesis a presión (hidrógeno, anhídrido carbónico y monóxido de carbono). Según las proyecciones, la capacidad mundial se elevaría a 30 millones de toneladas en 1995.

El metanol se utiliza en la producción industrial de numerosos compuestos orgánicos importantes, sobre todo metil terbutil éter (MTBE), formaldehído, ácido acético, éteres de metilglicol, metilamina, haluros de metilo y metacrilato de metilo.

El metanol es un elemento constitutivo de un gran número de disolventes y productos de consumo disponibles en el comercio, como pinturas, gomas laca, barnices, diluyentes de pinturas, soluciones limpiadoras, soluciones anticongelantes, líquidos limpiaparabrisas y anticongelantes para automóviles, líquidos de multicopista, desnaturalizante para el etanol y pegamento para actividades de pasatiempo y artesanía. Una aplicación potencialmente en gran escala del metanol está en su uso directo como combustible, mezclado con gasolina o para aumentar su volumen. Hay que señalar que la mayor morbilidad y mortalidad se ha relacionado con la ingestión oral deliberada o accidental de mezclas con contenidos de metanol.

Se ha detectado metanol en los gases de escape de motores tanto de gasolina como diésel y en el humo del tabaco.

3. Niveles ambientales y exposición humana

Las emisiones de metanol se derivan principalmente de los diversos usos industriales y domésticos como disolvente, su producción, la manufactura final y las pérdidas durante el almacenamiento a granel y la manipulación.

Pueden darse exposiciones al metanol en los lugares de trabajo mediante inhalación o contacto cutáneo. Muchos de los límites nacionales de exposición para la higiene del trabajo parecen indicar que los trabajadores están protegidos de cualquier efecto adverso si la exposición no supera un promedio ponderado por el tiempo de 260 mg/m^3 (200 ppm) de metanol en cualquier jornada de trabajo de 8 horas y en una semana laboral de 40 horas.

La exposición general actual de la población por medio del aire es normalmente 10 000 veces inferior a los límites ocupacionales. La población general está expuesta al metanol en el aire a concentraciones que oscilan entre menos de 0,001 mg/m^3 (0,8 ppm) en el aire del medio rural y cerca de 0,04 mg/m^3 (30 ppm) en el aire urbano.

Los datos sobre la presencia del metanol en el agua potable de uso inmediato son limitados, pero con frecuencia se encuentra metanol en efluentes industriales.

En el caso de que el uso previsto del metanol como combustible alternativo o mezclado con otros combustibles aumente considerablemente, cabe prever que habrá una exposición generalizada al metanol por medio de la inhalación de vapores procedentes de los vehículos que funcionen con él y del bombeo o la absorción percutánea de combustibles o mezclas de metanol.

4. Distribución y transformación en el medio ambiente

El metanol se degrada fácilmente en el medio ambiente mediante procesos de fotooxidación y biodegradación. Se han descrito semividas de 7-18 días para la reacción atmosférica del metanol con radicales oxhidrilo.

Hay muchos géneros y cepas de microorganismos capaces de utilizar el metanol como sustrato de crecimiento. El metanol es fácilmente degradable en condiciones tanto aerobias como anaerobias en una amplia variedad de medios naturales, entre ellos agua dulce y salada, sedimentos y suelos, agua freática, material de acuíferos y aguas residuales industriales; el 70% del metanol de los alcantarillados se suele degradar en un plazo de 5 días.

El metanol es un sustrato de crecimiento normal de muchos microorganismos del suelo, que son capaces de degradarlo completamente a anhídrido carbónico y agua.

El metanol tiene una capacidad de absorción bastante baja en los suelos. La bioconcentración en la mayoría de los organismos es escasa.

El metanol es poco tóxico para los organismos acuáticos y terrestres y no es probable que se observen efectos debidos a su exposición en el medio ambiente, excepto en el caso de un derrame.

5. Absorción, distribución, biotransformación y eliminación

El metanol se absorbe fácilmente por inhalación, ingestión y exposición cutánea y se distribuye rápidamente en los tejidos siguiendo la distribución del agua corporal. Por los pulmones y los riñones se excreta una pequeña cantidad de metanol sin cambios.

Tras la digestión se alcanzan niveles máximos en suero en un plazo de 30-90 minutos, y se reparte por todo el organismo con un volumen de distribución aproximado de 0,6 litros/kg.

El metanol se metaboliza principalmente en el hígado siguiendo una fase oxidativa secuencial a formaldehído, ácido fórmico y anhídrido carbónico. El paso inicial consiste en la oxidación a formaldehído por acción de la alcohol deshidrogenasa hepática, que es un proceso saturable limitante de la velocidad. La afinidad relativa de la alcohol deshidrogenasa por el etanol y el metanol es aproximadamente de 20:1. En el segundo paso, el formaldehído se oxida por acción de la formaldehído deshidrogenasa a ácido fórmico o formiato, en función del pH. En el tercer paso, el ácido fórmico se destoxifica a anhídrido carbónico mediante reacciones dependientes del folato.

La eliminación del metanol de la sangre a través de la orina y el aire exhalado y por el metabolismo parece ser lenta en todas las especies, especialmente si se compara con el etanol. En el proceso se han descrito períodos de semieliminación de 24 horas o más con dosis superiores a 1 g/kg y de 2,5-3 horas para dosis inferiores a 0,1 g/kg. El ritmo de desintoxicación metabólica o eliminación del formiato sí es muy distinto entre los roedores y los primates, constituyendo la base de las enormes diferencias de toxicidad del metanol observadas entre ambos grupos.

6.   Efectos en mamíferos de laboratorio y en sistemas de ensayo *in vitro*

6.1   *Toxicidad sistémica*

La toxicidad aguda y a corto plazo del metanol varía mucho entre las distintas especies, siendo máxima en las especies con una capacidad relativamente escasa para metabolizar el formiato. En tales casos de metabolismo deficiente del formiato, se produce una intoxicación letal por metanol como consecuencia de la acidosis metabólica y la toxicidad neuronal, mientras que en los animales que metabolizan fácilmente el formiato la muerte suele deberse a las consecuencias de la depresión del sistema nervioso central (coma, insuficiencia respiratoria, etc.). En las especies de primates sensibles (el ser humano y los monos) aumenta la concentración del formiato en sangre tras la exposición al metanol, pero no en los roedores, los conejos y los perros resistentes. Los primates humanos y no humanos tienen una sensibilidad única a los efectos tóxicos del metanol. En conjunto, el metanol tiene una toxicidad aguda baja para los animales no primates. Los valores de la DL_{50} y las dosis letales mínimas tras la exposición oral oscilan entre 7000 y 13 000 mg/kg en ratas, ratones, conejos y perros y entre 2000 y 7000 mg/kg en el mono.

Las ratas expuestas a concentraciones de metanol de hasta 6500 mg/m^3 (5000 ppm) 6 horas al día y 5 días a la semana durante un período de 4 semanas no mostraron ningún efecto relacionado con la exposición, salvo el aumento de la exudación alrededor de la nariz y de los ojos. Se consideró que esto era un reflejo de la irritación de las vías respiratorias superiores.

Las ratas expuestas a concentraciones de vapor de metanol de hasta 13 000 mg/m^3 (10 000 ppm) 6 horas al día y 5 días a la semana durante un período de 6 semanas, no mostraron ninguna toxicidad pulmonar.

En el conejo el metanol es moderadamente irritante de los ojos. En una prueba de maximización modificada no se produjo sensibilización cutánea.

Entre los efectos tóxicos observados en primates expuestos al metanol cabe mencionar la acidosis metabólica y la toxicidad ocular, pero estos efectos no aparecen normalmente en roedores con una concentración suficiente de folato. Las diferencias de toxicidad se deben a variaciones en la tasa del metabolismo del formiato, metabolito del metanol. Por ejemplo, la eliminación del formiato de la sangre de los primates expuestos es como mínimo un 50% más lenta que en los roedores.

En monos que recibieron dosis de metanol superiores a 3000 mg/kg con sonda se observó ataxia, debilidad y letargo a las pocas horas de exposición. Estos signos mostraron una tendencia a desaparecer en un plazo de 24 horas y los siguió un coma transitorio en algunos de los animales.

En monos expuestos a metanol durante 6 horas al día y 5 días a la semana, con 20 exposiciones repetidas a 6500 mg/m^3 (5000 ppm) de metanol no aparecieron efectos oculares.

6.2 Genotoxicidad y carcinogenicidad

El metanol ha dado resultados negativos en cuanto a la mutación genética en ensayos con bacterias y levaduras, pero indujo anomalías en la segregación cromosómica en *Aspergillus*. No indujo intercambios de cromátidas hermanas en células de hámster chino *in vitro*, pero provocó un aumento considerable de la frecuencia de las mutaciones en células de linfoma de ratón L5178Y.

La inhalación de metanol no indujo daños en los cromosomas de ratones. Hay algunas pruebas de que la administración oral e intraperitoneal ha aumentado la incidencia de daños en los cromosomas de ratones.

No hay ninguna prueba en estudios con animales que indique que el metanol es carcinógeno, aunque se reconoce que se carece de un modelo animal apropiado.

6.3 Toxicidad reproductiva, embriotoxicidad y teratogenicidad

Se han descrito resultados contradictorios en relación con los efectos de la inhalación de metanol durante un período de hasta 6 semanas sobre las concentraciones de gonadotropina y testosterona.

La inhalación de metanol por roedores gestantes durante todo el período de la embriogénesis induce una amplia variedad de efectos teratogénicos y embrioletales dependientes de la concentración. En fetos de ratas expuestas 7 horas al día durante 7-15 días de gestación a 26 000 mg/m^3 (20 000 ppm) de metanol se encontraron malformaciones relacionadas con el tratamiento, predominantemente costillas cervicales adicionales o rudimentarias y defectos del aparato urinario o cardiovascular. Con este nivel de exposición se observó una ligera toxicidad materna, pero no se detectó ningún efecto adverso para la madre o la descendencia en animales expuestos a 6500 mg/m^3 (5000 ppm), lo cual se interpretó como la concentración sin efectos adversos observados (NOAEL) para este sistema de prueba.

Se registró una mayor incidencia de exencefalia y paladar hendido en la descendencia de ratones CD-1 expuestos 7 horas al día durante los días 6-15 de gestación a concentraciones de metanol de 6500 mg/m^3 (5000 ppm) o más. La mortalidad embriofetal aumentó a concentraciones de 9825 mg/m^3 (7500 ppm) o más y fue mayor la incidencia de resorciones de toda la descendencia. A concentraciones de 13 000 y 19 500 mg/m^3 (10 000 y 15 000 ppm) se observó un peso fetal reducido. La NOAEL para la toxicidad del desarrollo fue de 1300 mg/m^3 (1000 ppm) de metanol. No se encontraron pruebas de toxicidad materna en la exposición a concentraciones de metanol inferiores a 9000 mg/m^3 (7000 ppm).

Cuando se administraron mediante sonda 4 g/kg de metanol a la descendencia de ratones CD-1 gestantes, la incidencia de los efectos adversos en la resorción, los defectos externos como el paladar hendido y el peso del feto fue análoga a la observada en el grupo expuesto por inhalación a 13 000 mg/m^3 (10 000 ppm), posiblemente debido al mayor ritmo de respiración del ratón. Éste es más sensible que la rata a la toxicidad en el desarrollo provocada por el metanol inhalado.

En hembras CD-1 expuestas a 19 500 mg/m^3 (15 000 ppm) durante 6 horas diarias a lo largo de la organogénesis (días de gestación 6-15) aparecieron signos neurológicos transitorios y una reducción del peso corporal. Entre las malformaciones fetales registradas con 13 000 y 19 500 mg/m^3 (10 000 y 15 000 ppm) cabe mencionar defectos neurales y oculares, paladar hendido, hidronefrosis y anomalías de las extremidades.

7.   Efectos en el ser humano

El ser humano y los primates no humanos tienen una sensibilidad única a la intoxicación por metanol, caracterizándose los efectos tóxicos en estas especies por acidemia fórmica, acidosis metabólica, toxicidad ocular, depresión del sistema nervioso, ceguera, coma y la muerte. Casi toda la información disponible sobre la toxicidad del metanol en el ser humano se refiere a las consecuencias de exposiciones agudas más que crónicas. La inmensa mayoría de las intoxicaciones por metanol se han debido al consumo de bebidas adulteradas y de productos con metanol. Aunque la ingestión es con diferencia la vía más frecuente de intoxicación, la inhalación de concentraciones elevadas de vapor de metanol o la absorción percutánea de líquidos metanólicos son tan eficaces como la vía oral para la producción de efectos tóxicos agudos. La consecuencia más conocida para la salud de una exposición a plazo más largo a niveles inferiores de metanol es una amplia gama de efectos oculares.

Las propiedades tóxicas del metanol se basan en factores que rigen tanto su conversión en ácido fórmico como el posterior metabolismo del formiato a anhídrido carbónico en la ruta del folato. La toxicidad es manifiesta si la generación de formiato continúa a un ritmo superior al del metabolismo.

No se conoce con seguridad la dosis letal del metanol para el ser humano. La dosis letal mínima del metanol en ausencia de tratamiento médico está comprendida entre 0,3 y 1 g/kg. No se conoce la dosis mínima que provoca defectos visuales permanentes.

La gravedad de la acidosis metabólica es variable y puede no tener correlación con la cantidad de metanol ingerido. Una característica destacada de la intoxicación aguda por metanol es la enorme variabilidad interindividual de la dosis tóxica.

Parece que dos factores determinantes importantes de la susceptibilidad humana a la toxicidad por metanol son: 1) ingestión junto con etanol, que reduce el ritmo de entrada de metanol en la ruta metabólica, y 2) la situación del folato hepático, que rige la tasa de desintoxicación del formiato.

Los síntomas y signos de intoxicación por metanol, que pueden aparecer solo transcurrido un período asintomático aproximado de 12 a 24 horas, son perturbaciones visuales, náuseas, dolor abdominal y muscular, mareo, debilidad y perturbaciones de la conciencia que van desde el coma hasta las convulsiones clónicas. Las alteraciones visuales aparecen en general entre las 12 y las 48 horas después de la ingestión del metanol y van desde la ligera fotofobia y la visión brumosa o borrosa hasta una reducción acentuada de la agudeza visual y la ceguera completa. En casos extremos se produce la muerte. La principal característica clínica es una acidosis metabólica grave del tipo de deficiencia de aniones. La acidosis se atribuye en gran medida al ácido fórmico producido al metabolizarse el metanol.

La concentración normal en sangre de metanol procedente de fuentes endógenas es de menos de 0,5 mg/litro (0,02 mmol/litro), pero las fuentes alimenticias pueden elevarla. En general aparecen efectos en el sistema nervioso central cuando la concentración de metanol en sangre supera los 200 mg/litro (6 mmol/litro); se detectan síntomas oculares por encima de 500 mg/litros (16 mmol/litro) y se han registrado casos de letalidad en pacientes no tratados con concentraciones iniciales de metanol del orden de 1500-2000 mg/litro (47-62 mmol/litro).

La inhalación aguda de concentraciones de vapor de metanol por debajo de 260 mg/m^3 o la ingestión de cantidades de hasta 20 mg/kg de metanol por parte de personas sanas o con una deficiencia moderada de folato no debe dar lugar a la acumulación de formiato por encima de las concentraciones endógenas.

Se ha informado de alteraciones visuales de varios tipos (visión borrosa, reducción del campo visivo, cambios en la percepción de los colores y ceguera temporal o permanente) en trabajadores expuestos a concentraciones de metanol en el aire de alrededor de 1500 mg/m^3 (1200 ppm) o más.

Un límite muy utilizado de exposición en el trabajo para el metanol es el de 260 mg/m^3 (200 ppm), concebido para proteger a los trabajadores de cualquiera de los efectos de la acidosis metabólica por ácido fórmico inducida por el metanol y de la toxicidad ocular y del sistema nervioso.

No se ha notificado ningún otro efecto adverso del metanol en el ser humano, salvo una ligera irritación cutánea y ocular con exposiciones muy superiores a los 26 mg/m^3 (200 ppm).

8. Efectos en los organismos del medio ambiente

Los valores de la CL_{50} en organismos acuáticos oscilan entre 1300 y 15 900 mg/litro para los invertebrados (48 y 96 horas de exposición) y entre 13 000 y 29 000 mg/litro para los peces (96 horas de exposición).

El metanol es poco tóxico para los organismos acuáticos siendo poco probable la observación de efectos debidos a exposición ambiental al metanol, excepto en el caso de un derrame.

---

[a]   Out of print